ANCIENT TECHNOLOGY

ANCIENT MEDICINE

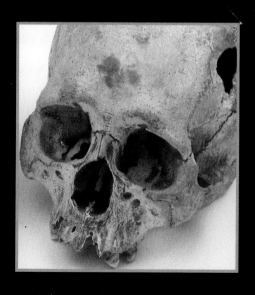

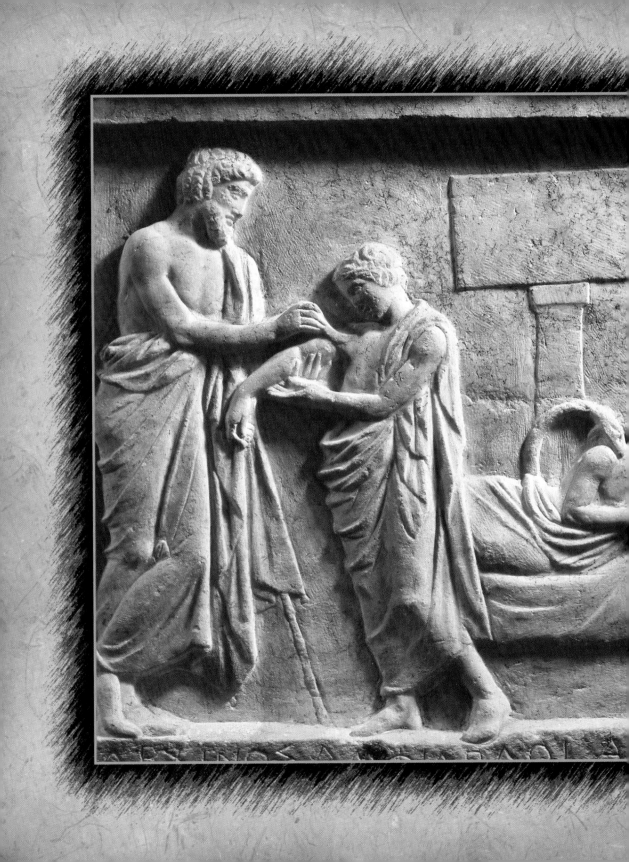

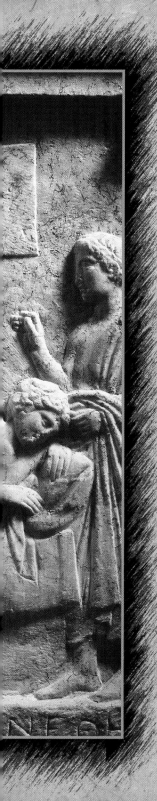

ANCIENT TECHNOLOGY

ANCIENT MEDICINE

FROM SORCERY TO SURGERY

by Michael Woods
and
Mary B. Woods

RP RUNESTONE PRESS • MINNEAPOLIS
A DIVISION OF LERNER PUBLISHING GROUP

Dedicated to John Robinson Block who, like his father, Paul Block Jr., encouraged efforts to increase public understanding of science and technology.

Series designer: Zachary Marell
Series editors: Joelle E. Riley and Dina Drits
Copy editor: Margaret J. Goldstein
Photograph researcher: Dan Mesnik

Runestone Press
A Division of Lerner Publishing Group
241 First Avenue North
Minneapolis, MN 55401 U.S.A.

Website address: www.lernerbooks.com

LIBRARY OF CONGRESS CATALOGING-IN-PUBLICATION DATA

Woods, Michael, 1946–
    Ancient medicine : from sorcery to surgery / Michael Woods and
Mary B. Woods.
        p.   cm. — (Ancient technology)
    Includes bibliographical references and index.
    Summary: Describes medical techniques such as brain surgery,
splints, taking a pulse, forceps, and sanitation in ancient
civilizations including the Stone Age, Egypt, Greece, China, India,
and Rome.
    ISBN 0–8225–2992–0 (alk. paper)
    1. Medicine, Ancient—Juvenile literature. 2. Medical technology—
History—Juvenile literature. [1. Medicine, Ancient. 2. Medical
technology.] I. Woods, Mary B. (Mary Boyle), 1946–. II. Title.
III. Series.
R135.W73 2000
610'.9'01—dc21   98–36124

Manufactured in the United States of America
1 2 3 4 5 6 – JR – 05 04 03 02 01 00

TABLE OF CONTENTS

Introduction / 6

Chapter 1, The Stone Age / 11

Chapter 2, Ancient Egypt / 21

Chapter 3, Ancient India / 33

Chapter 4, Ancient China / 45

Chapter 5, Ancient Greece / 53

Chapter 6, Ancient Rome / 69

Glossary / 84

Bibliography / 85

Index / 86

What do you think of when you hear the word *technology?* You probably think of something totally new. You might think of research laboratories filled with computers, powerful microscopes, and other scientific tools. But technology doesn't refer to just brand-new machines and discoveries. Technology is as old as humankind.

Technology is the use of knowledge, inventions, and discoveries to make human life better. The word *technology* comes from two Greek words. One, *tekhne,* means "art" or "craft." The other, *logos,* means "word" or "speech." The ancient Greeks originally used the word *technology* to mean a discussion of arts and crafts. But, in modern times, *technology* usually refers to a craft, technique, or tool itself.

People use many kinds of technology. Farming is one kind of technology. Transportation and construction are also kinds of technology. These technologies and many others help make human life easier, safer, and more enjoyable. This book takes a look at another important kind of technology—one that has helped human life tremendously. That technology is medicine.

ANCIENT ROOTS

You've probably heard people remark, "There's nothing new under the sun!" That's often true when we're talking about medical technology. Modern medical researchers rarely make a discovery that is totally new. Most medical breakthroughs are only tiny advances—just small steps along the road to treating or curing a disease. That road often began thousands of years ago.

Indeed, much of modern technology has ancient roots. Scientists who lived thousands of years ago built many of the foundations of modern technology. These scientists gave us ideas and knowledge, and we improved on them.

The word *ancient* refers to a time period beginning with the first humans on earth and ending with the fall of the Western Roman Empire in A.D. 476. The first human beings lived about 2.5 million years ago. One of the traits that archaeologists—scientists who study the remains of past societies—use to distinguish human beings from their prehuman ancestors is the use of technology, or tools. The first technology was primitive, involving the use of simple stone tools. Nevertheless, it was technology.

TECHNOLOGY'S SPREAD

No country's technology develops in isolation. Ancient peoples had a lot of contact with one another. The ancient Greeks, for instance, shipped pottery, marble, olive oil, wool, wine, and other products to countries all around the Mediterranean Sea. Their ships did not return home empty. Instead, they brought glass and grain from Egypt, dyes from Phoenicia, copper from Cyprus. Ancient

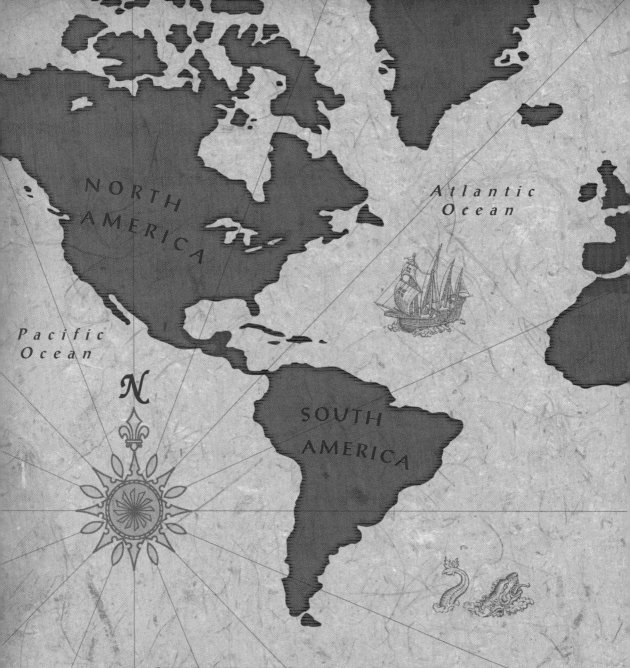

CIVILIZATIONS OF THE
Ancient World
(through A.D. 476)

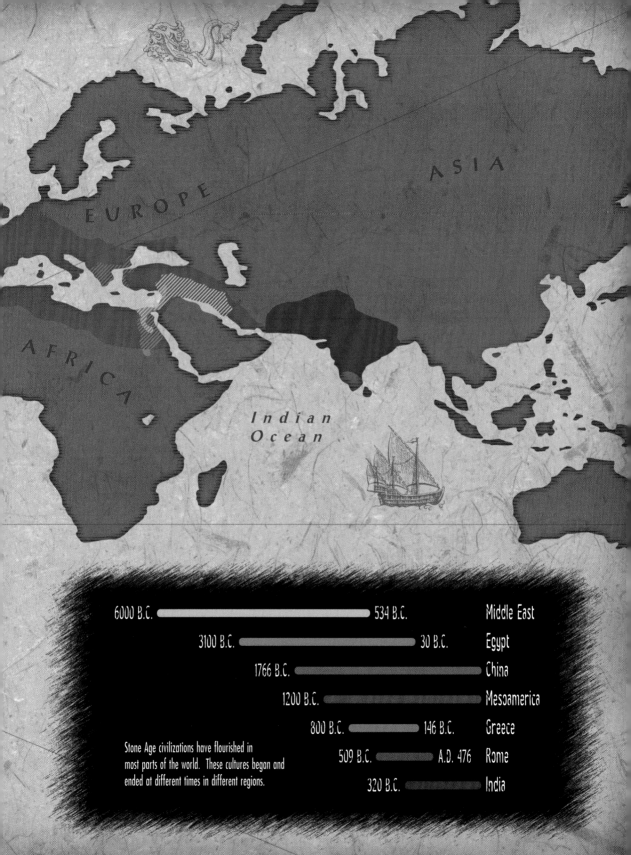

EUROPE

ASIA

AFRICA

*Indian
Ocean*

6000 B.C. ▬▬▬▬▬▬ 534 B.C.		Middle East
3100 B.C. ▬▬▬▬▬ 30 B.C.		Egypt
1766 B.C. ▬▬▬▬		China
1200 B.C. ▬▬▬		Mesoamerica
800 B.C. ▬▬ 146 B.C.		Greece
509 B.C. ▬ A.D. 476		Rome
320 B.C. ▬▬		India

Stone Age civilizations have flourished in
most parts of the world. These cultures began and
ended at different times in different regions.

traders also exchanged knowledge. From Phoenicia, the Greeks borrowed an alphabet. From Egypt, they learned geometry and how to apply it in construction.

Wars also led to the exchange of technology and knowledge among cultures. When the ancient Greeks conquered the Minoans around 1450 B.C., they obtained medical technology, including drugs, surgical procedures, and new ways of treating and diagnosing disease.

A LOT WITH A LITTLE

Ancient doctors did not have powerful computers and microscopes. They did not have drugstores full of tablets, creams, and antibiotics for treating patients. But they had just as much curiosity and creativity as modern medical researchers. With very few tools to help them, ancient physicians accomplished great things.

For instance, ancient doctors derived medicines from the bark, flowers, stems, leaves, and roots of plants. Many of these remedies are still used. Stone Age doctors performed brain surgery—eight thousand years ago! Ancient Indian doctors performed plastic surgery. Roman doctors performed eye surgery to fix cataracts.

Ancient doctors left a rich legacy of medical knowledge and technology. This book tells the story of these contributions. Read on if you love surprises and the adventure of discovery. But beware! You'll also encounter a lot of blood and guts!

chapter **1** one

THE STONE AGE

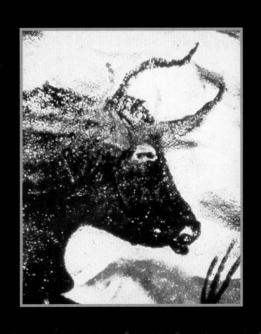

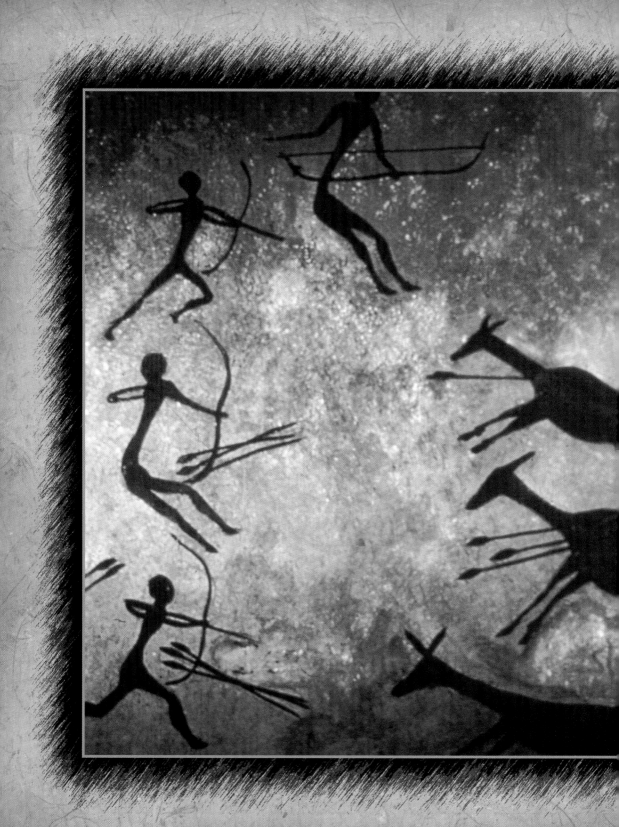

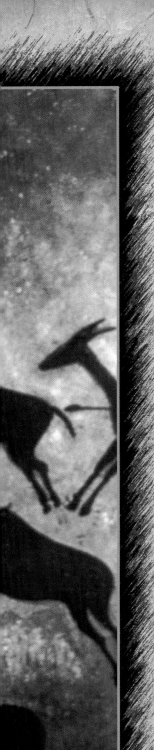

Cave painting of a deer hunt, Castellón, Spain

n 1867, a famous French physician named Paul Broca ran his hands over a four-thou-sand-year-old skull sent to his laboratory in Paris by an archaeologist. Someone had cut a big chunk of bone from the skull. Dr. Broca squinted and frowned as he inspected the hole. The archaeologist thought that some Stone Age barbarian had killed an enemy, then cut the hole to make a horrible drinking cup. As evidence, he noted that bone at the edge of the hole had been carefully polished so that people could drink without cutting their lips on the sharp edges of bone. Did Dr. Broca agree?

Dr. Broca was the world's greatest brain surgeon. Part of your brain, Broca's area, is named in his honor. But he never had seen anything to match the drinking cup skull. Dr. Broca quickly realized that the polish on the edges of the cut actually was new bone tissue. As bone heals after an injury, fresh tissue grows in the cracks and pores. That growth results in a smooth, shiny appearance.

13

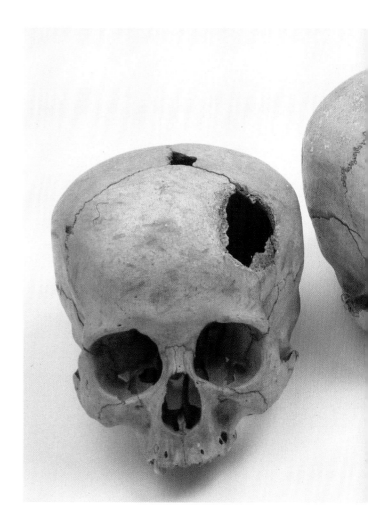

Four-thousand-year-old trepanned skulls found in Peru

There could be no doubt. The hole had been made in the skull of a living person, not a dead one. The skull actually belonged to a patient who had undergone brain surgery in the Stone Age! And the patient had lived long enough, probably months, for the bone to begin healing. Dr. Broca even knew the name of the operation, trepanation. This procedure involves cutting or drilling an opening in the skull

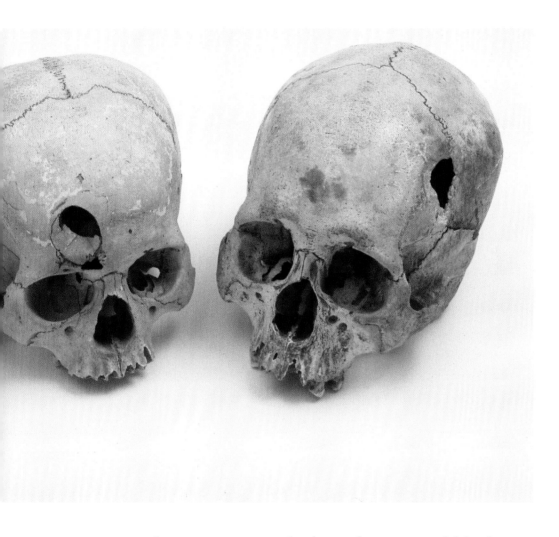

to relieve pressure on the brain from internal bleeding or other problems.

Physicians seldom dared to perform such surgery in the 1860s. Procedures such as trepanation usually resulted in fatal brain infections. At the best hospitals in London and Paris, three out of four brain surgery patients died. Yet this Stone Age patient had undergone brain surgery and lived!

Since Broca's time, archaeologists have uncovered hundreds of other ancient skulls showing the same clear evidence of brain surgery. The oldest known trepanned skull was uncovered from a grave in southern France. It dates from about eight thousand years ago. Other trepanned skulls have been traced to Stone Age people in the Middle East, India, China, and Peru.

When studying trepanned skulls, archaeologists look for the "polished" edges that indicate bone regrowth. These edges show that the patient survived surgery and lived long enough to heal. Some studies indicate that three out of four ancient patients survived. In some skulls, healing is extensive. These patients must have lived for years after surgery.

What diseases did ancient brain surgeons hope to cure with trepanation, the first known surgical treatment? Modern doctors know that trepanation can relieve a buildup of pressure inside the skull—perhaps caused by bleeding from a severe blow to the head. Did Stone Age people recognize that trepanation could relieve excess pressure on the brain? Archaeologists don't think so.

EVIL SPIRITS IN THE HEAD

The Stone Age was a period before written history. Stone Age peoples used simple tools made from stone. Archaeologists often divide the Stone Age into two parts. The Old Stone Age, or Paleolithic period, began around 500,000 B.C. and lasted until about 10,000 B.C. The New Stone Age, or Neolithic period, lasted from about 10,000 B.C. to about 3500 B.C. Archaeologists have found remains of Stone Age cultures in China, Africa, Europe, Asia, the Middle East, and other parts of the world.

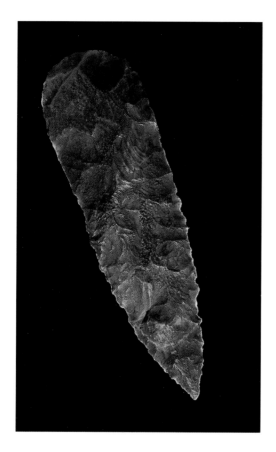

Razor-sharp flint spearhead made in the late Neolithic period

Since there are no written records from the Stone Age, archaeologists study skeletons, stone tools, paintings, and other artifacts to learn about Stone Age cultures. They also study records of other primitive societies, such as the Australian Aborigines, that lasted into modern times.

Archaeologists know that medicine in the Stone Age was based not on science but on magic and superstition. Instead of physicians, Stone Age people turned to medicine men and women, witch doctors, sorcerers, and shamans, who were believed to have supernatural powers.

Stone Age people did not have scientific explanations for natural events. For instance, they most likely thought that thunder, lightning, wind, rain, and snow were willed by supernatural beings. If a child became sick, its parents may have believed it was because someone—perhaps an enemy—had willed the sickness. If someone developed severe headaches, seizures, or strange behavior, evil spirits were probably responsible. Many archaeologists think that trepanation began as a superstitious ritual to release these evil spirits from the head.

Stone Age people were skilled in the production of stone knives and drills. Don't scoff at the idea of using stone instruments for brain surgery. Archaeologists know that knives made from obsidian, a volcanic glass, were razor sharp. Stone Age hunters could butcher a mammoth in minutes with these tools. Drills made from a bow and a fire-hardened wooden shaft could cut through bone. People worked the drills by looping the bowstring around the shaft, then pulling the bow back and forth to rotate the shaft.

SPLINTS FOR BROKEN BONES

One scientist who studied bones from Stone Age skeletons discovered that 53.8 percent of fractured leg and arm bones showed signs of healing. Indeed, the bones had healed so well that he concluded that Stone Age people knew how to splint fractures.

We can almost imagine the discovery. For years, an ancient medicine man or medicine woman observed hunters who were brought back to camp with broken legs. They lay near the fire for weeks, the slightest movement causing screams of agony. When finally able to stand, the hunters found themselves crippled. Their broken bones had healed so that one leg was shorter than the other.

After years of watching, the healer realized how to keep a broken leg from curling up and shortening: tie it to a stick so the bone stays straight. The medicine man or woman tried the new approach on the next patient. After a few months, the splinted bone healed to normal length. Many other early medical innovations probably occurred in the same way—by observation and experimentation.

STONE AGE DRUGS

Archaeologists know that prehistoric people fell victim to accidents, battle wounds, and conditions that caused severe pain. The marks of such conditions—infected teeth, gum disease, and arthritis—appear in ancient human bones. Did Stone Age people have anesthetics, or painkillers, to ease the pain of brain surgery, bone fractures, and other injuries? Did they have medicines for other diseases?

In fact, experts believe, early humans had surprisingly effective drugs. For instance, ancient people used plants from the nightshade family to relieve pain. Modern physicians know that some plants in this family are sources of powerful painkilling drugs such as scopolamine and atropine. But early people didn't know about these ingredients.

Ancient people probably discovered drugs by chance. People ate figs, for instance, because they were sweet. But those who ate too many figs got diarrhea. Maybe that's how people first discovered laxatives—some of the most important medicines in ancient times. Ancient people observed the effects of plants such as figs and passed their knowledge on from generation to generation.

Stone Age people probably discovered other treatments, such as massage and the use of pressure to stop bleeding, by instinct. When we feel pain, instinct tells us, "Rub." When we cut a finger, our first reaction is to grab and squeeze. The pressure squeezes blood vessels in the finger and stops the bleeding. Warmth eases aching joints and muscles, and ancient people may have used hot stones for this purpose.

Trepanation is one of the few bits of concrete evidence we have about Stone Age medical technology. It is astounding to think that doctors in 6000 B.C. were better brain surgeons than those of Dr. Broca's time—the relatively modern nineteenth century. Stone Age people almost certainly passed on to the groups that followed—the Egyptians, Greeks, and Romans—a rich heritage of other medical technology.

2

ANCIENT EGYPT

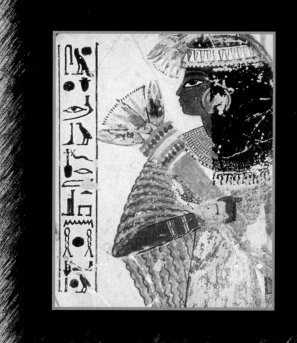

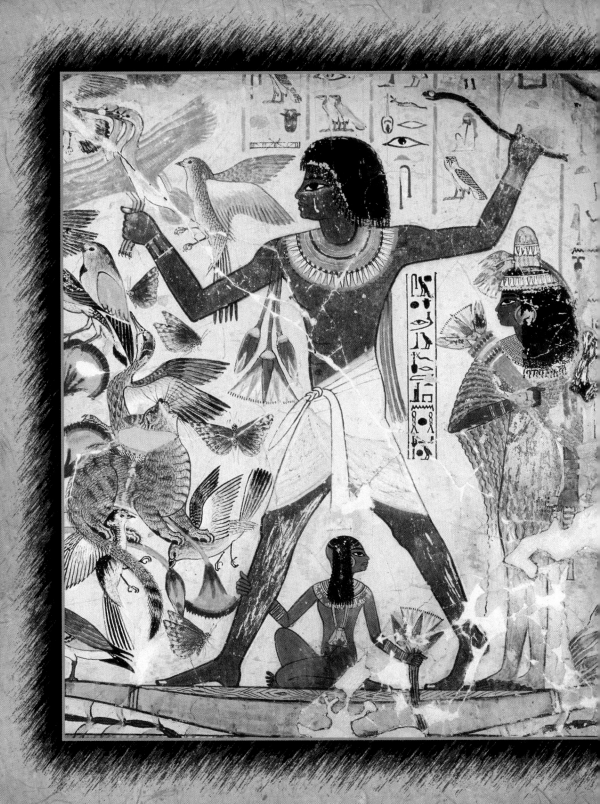

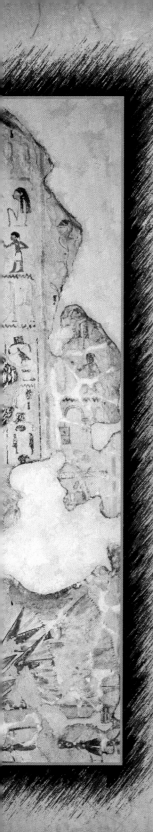

Painting on limestone from the tomb of
Nebamun at Thebes, Egypt

The first written accounts of ancient medical technology come from Egypt. Unlike Stone Age peoples, the Egyptians kept written records. Archaeologists use the word *civilization* (from the Latin *civitas*, or "city") to refer to groups such as the Egyptians who had systems of government, religion, social class, labor, and record keeping.

While we have little evidence about how Stone Age people treated diseases, the ancient Egyptians left detailed medical records, almost like modern textbooks. These records were written on long scrolls of papyrus, a kind of paper made from reeds. Some of the scrolls are several yards long, with writing on both sides. Ancient Egyptians used a type of picture-writing called hieroglyphics.

Archaeologists have found several medical papyruses in ancient tombs. The most important are the Kahun Papyrus, the Edwin H. Smith Papyrus, and the Ebers Papyrus. The Kahun Papyrus was written around 1900 B.C.

23

and deals with gynecology (women's health care) and childbirth. The Smith Papyrus, written about 1600 B.C., deals with surgery and the treatment of injuries. The Ebers Papyrus, written around 1550 B.C., is the most famous of all. Found between the legs of a body in a tomb near Thebes, it is an ancient medical encyclopedia. It contains instructions for diagnosing and treating diseases and wounds, prescriptions for many medications, descriptions of how the heart and other organs function, and other information.

THE FIRST KNOWN PHYSICIAN

For thousands of years, ancient people treated themselves and their families, or relied on magicians or healers with no formal medical training. Healers probably spent most of their time farming or tending flocks. They worked at medicine part-time, only when called to an illness or injury. It was a great advance when medicine became a full-time occupation.

Who was the world's first physician? Sir William Osler (1849–1919), a Canadian doctor, awarded the honor to an Egyptian named Imhotep. Dr. Osler wrote that Imhotep was "the first figure of a physician to stand out clearly from the mists of antiquity." Images of Imhotep have appeared on commemorative postage stamps and in medical schools and clinics. The senior class yearbook at the Boston University School of Medicine is named *The Imhotepian.*

Imhotep was born around 2650 B.C. in Memphis, near modern Cairo. His name means "he who comes in peace." Imhotep was chancellor, or chief executive assistant, to the pharaoh Zoser. He also designed the first pyramid in Egypt—and probably the first in the world—the Step Pyra-

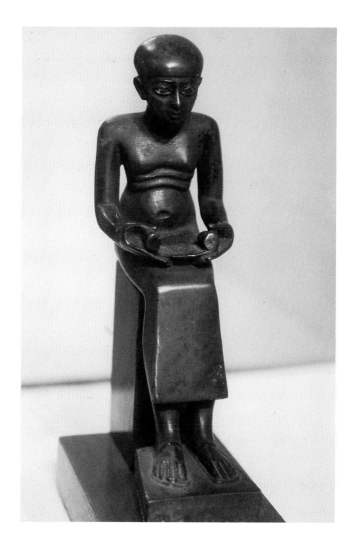

Imhotep, the founder of Egyptian medicine

mid at Saqqara. The Egyptians later worshiped Imhotep as a god. Much of Imhotep's fame rests on his work as an architect and engineer, not as a doctor. In fact, there is little evidence that Imhotep actually treated people.

Hesy Re is another candidate for first physician. He lived in Egypt around 2600 B.C. and served as "Chief of Physicians and Dentists to the Pyramid Builders." Hesy Re and Imhotep may have known each other. Stone inscriptions indicate that Hesy Re performed an early form of oral surgery. He drilled holes into a patient's gum near an abscessed, or badly infected, tooth. This procedure allowed pus to drain and would have relieved the patient's excruciating pain.

AHEAD OF THE REST

People throughout the ancient world thought that Egypt had the best medical care. Kings and princes of other countries wrote to the pharaoh, asking that Egyptian physicians be sent to their courts. In *The Odyssey*, which was written in the eighth century B.C., the Greek poet Homer describes wonderful drugs that an Egyptian physician gave to Queen Helen of Sparta. Homer noted that "in medical knowledge the Egyptian leaves the rest of the world behind."

Not only did ancient Egypt have the first physicians but it also had the first specialists, doctors specially trained to treat diseases of individual parts of the body. The Greek historian Herodotus wrote:

> Medicine is thereby divided among the Egyptians so that each doctor knows but one disease and none of the others. All Egypt is stuffed with physicians. Some appoint themselves as experts on the eyes, others "do" the head, others teeth, others matters having to do with the belly, and others specialize in hidden diseases.

If you transliterate the ancient Egyptian word for physician into modern English, you wind up with the word *swnw* (possibly pronounced "soo-new" or "oor-soun-ou"). Some physicians had more elaborate titles. For instance, the

Egyptians called their version of the modern proctologist "The Shepherd of the Anus." He may have specialized in all diseases of the stomach or intestine.

Female doctors may have been common in ancient Egypt. A female physician named Peseshet lived in Egypt around 2500 B.C. She is the first female physician known by name. But Peseshet's title, "Lady Overseer of Lady Physicians," implies that she was one of many female doctors.

MRHT, BYT, AND FTT

Grease, honey, and lint. Those were the ingredients in one of ancient Egypt's most popular salves for cuts, scrapes, and other wounds. This ancient forerunner of triple antibiotic ointment really did work.

The grease might have been fat from an ox or ibis. It would have helped keep a bandage from sticking and tearing open a wound when the swnw changed a dressing. Although modern physicians don't recommend it, some people still put greasy salves such as petroleum jelly on minor burns and cuts.

Honey, modern scientists know, can destroy bacteria, which explains why honey doesn't spoil in beehives. One expert who tested this salve concluded that the Egyptians "happened to choose an ingredient that was practically harmless to the tissues, aseptic, antiseptic, and antibiotic . . . nothing else in ancient Egypt could have begun to match these properties of honey." Indeed, honey was an ingredient in more Egyptian medicines than any other substance.

Lint is fiber from cotton or another plant. The Egyptians often applied lint to cuts to stop the bleeding. Lint exhibits capillary action, meaning it will draw pus and other fluid out of a wound. Lint also would have helped bind together the other ingredients in Egyptian wound salve.

Egyptian Surgery

Egyptian doctors did little or no major surgery, which involves cutting deep into the body—perhaps because the Egyptians believed that the body must be kept intact for its journey into the afterlife. Egyptian doctors did perform minor surgical procedures, however, such as lancing boils and stitching up battle wounds. Another common procedure was circumcision, removal of the flap of skin at the end of the penis.

Modern physicians recognize that circumcision has health benefits: circumcised men are less apt to get certain diseases. The Egyptians and other ancient peoples recognized the importance of circumcision, too. The world's first known picture of a surgical operation, carved on the wall of an Egyptian tomb around 2250 B.C., shows doctors performing a circumcision.

Egyptian surgeons, such as those shown in the circumcision mural, had razor-sharp knives made from flint or obsidian. They also had surprisingly sharp "disposable" blades, made from the stems of dried reeds. Metal knives and instruments were in use by 1500 B.C.

A famous relief on the wall of the temple at Kom Ombo, built around A.D. 100, shows about 40 different medical instruments. These include speculums to open the vagina and rectum for internal examinations, scales for weighing medicines, containers for holding solid and liquid medicines, forceps, hooks for spreading open incisions and wounds, and curettes for scraping away infected tissue.

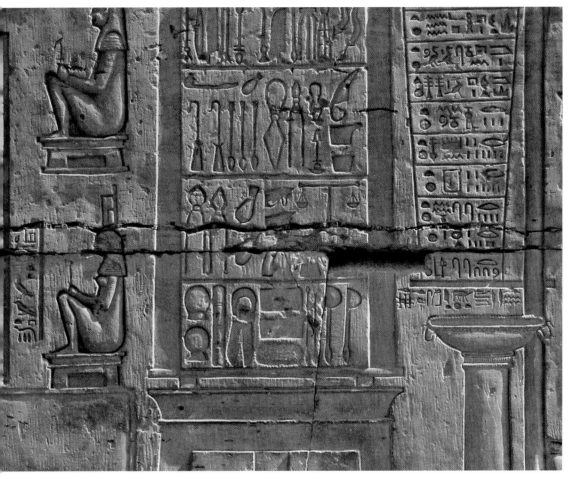

Wall relief from the Temple of Sobek and Horus at Kom Ombo, Egypt, showing a variety of surgical instruments

TOOTHISTS

Sand blew into everything in ancient Egypt; people often ate a mixture of food and sand. The grit acted like sandpaper, quickly wearing the hard coating of enamel off people's teeth and exposing the inner nerves and blood vessels.

People probably got horrible toothaches and abscesses in ancient Egypt.

Dentists, called "toothists" or "toothworkers," thus were important medical personnel. Egyptian dentists did not treat toothaches in the easiest way, by pulling the tooth. Instead they applied medicines to the tooth, and even tried magic spells. Studies of mummies—bodies preserved after death— indicate that tooth decay became a bigger and bigger problem as Egyptian civilization advanced, and people ate more sweets.

Studies of mummies also indicate that dentists knew how to treat a badly infected tooth. They drilled holes into the gum surrounding the tooth so that the pus could drain. This procedure also relieved pain. Dentists also tried to keep loose teeth from falling out. They wrapped fine gold wire around a loose tooth, then fastened the wire to an adjacent tooth.

BAKING SODA FOR FRESH BREATH

Baking soda, or sodium bicarbonate, was used as a tooth cleaner long before modern baking soda toothpastes became popular. In fact, the ancient Egyptians probably introduced baking soda as a tooth-care product more than four thousand years ago. To sweeten foul breath, Egyptian men and women chewed lumps of natron. This natural soda consists of sodium carbonate and sodium bicarbonate and is found in deposits throughout Egypt.

The Egyptians used elaborate mouth rinses, much like modern mouthwashes. One popular rinse was made of frankincense, goose fat, cumin, honey, and water. So far as we know, the Egyptians did not use toothbrushes. But, like other ancient people, they may have cleaned their teeth with the frayed ends of twigs.

DRUGS THAT WORKED . . .

Egyptians were known around the world for their skill in compounding, or mixing, drugs. The modern English word *chemistry* comes from the Greek *chemi*, which means "the Black Land"—the ancient name for Egypt.

Many important drugs date to ancient Egypt. These include castor oil and figs, used as laxatives; opium to relieve pain, stop diarrhea, and induce sleep; cannabis, or marijuana, to stimulate the appetite and reduce anxiety; aloe to treat skin conditions; and pomegranate to kill intestinal worms. Some of these drugs are still prescribed by modern physicians.

Like modern women, women in ancient times sometimes wanted to avoid becoming pregnant. Some of the first known recipes for contraceptives appear in the Kahun Papyrus. The prescriptions included pastes of strange materials such as crocodile dung and sour milk that were inserted into the vagina. Modern researchers have found that some of the ancient contraceptives, including sour milk and the gum of the acacia tree, might have worked.

. . . AND SOME THAT DIDN'T

Of course, many medicines and treatments from ancient Egypt did not work. For instance, the Egyptians used mice—sometimes dead, rotten mice—in medicines for toothache, earache, and other conditions. Sometimes, doctors simply put a dead mouse right onto an aching tooth or swollen gum. Sometimes they mashed the mouse into a paste and mixed it with other ingredients. In the 1920s, some physicians in rural England and other countries were still treating patients with medicines made from mice.

Ancient Egyptian physicians also developed the first known treatment for baldness. The Ebers Papyrus described how to "make the hair of a bald person grow: Fat of lion, fat of hippopotamus, fat of crocodile, fat of cat, fat of serpent, fat of ibex, are mixed together and the head of a bald person is anointed therewith."

Of course, modern physicians and dentists would never be tempted to try most ancient Egyptian medical techniques. But advances from ancient Egypt certainly did help patients—and improved the body of medical technology handed down to other civilizations.

ANCIENT INDIA

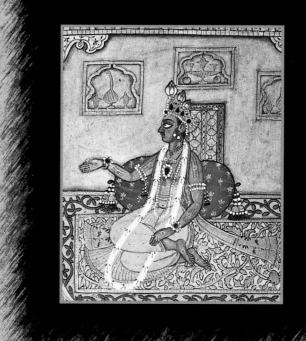

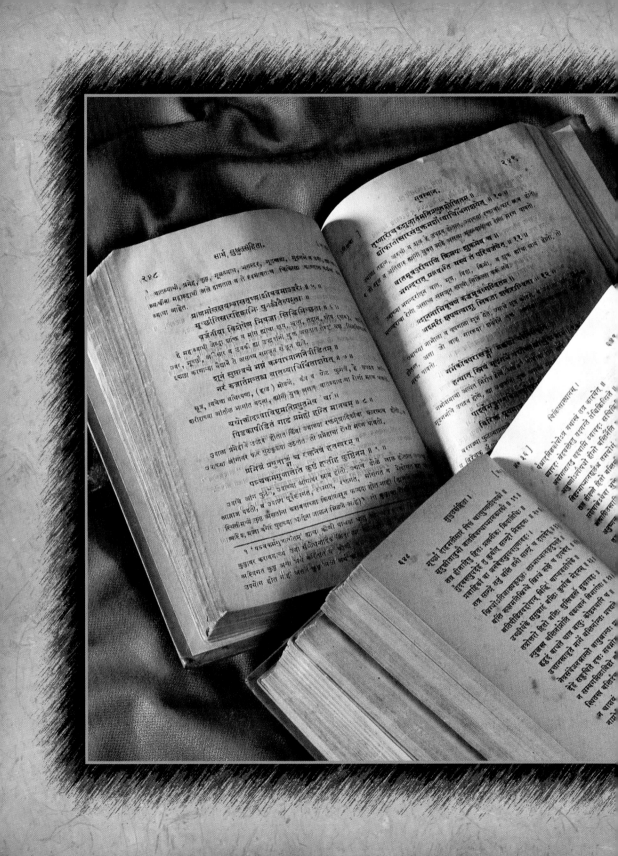

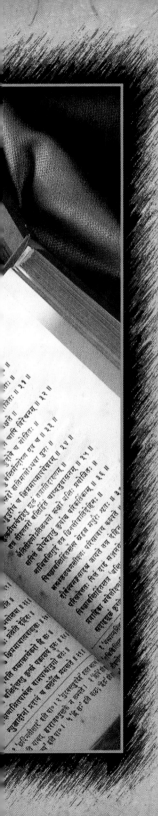

Modern copies of the *Sushruta Samhita,* a collection of ancient Indian medical writings

The earliest known Indian civilization emerged around 2500 B.C. in the Indus River Valley. It was home to great cities such as Mohenjo-Daro and Harappa. Around 1500 B.C., warlike nomads called Aryans swept in from the north. The Aryans conquered Indian cities and established traditions that lasted into modern times. They developed a caste system that divided Indian society into different classes, based in part on people's work. They also developed the Hindu religion and a written language called Sanskrit.

Ancient Indian, or Hindu, medicine was called *ayurveda,* which means "science of life" or "knowledge of life." The word for physician was *vaidya,* or "he who has wisdom." Much of our knowledge about ancient Hindu medicine comes from two collections of medical writings. One, the *Sushruta Samhita,* was written by a surgeon named Sushruta. The other, the *Charaka Samhita,* was written by a physician named Charaka. *Samhita* means "collection."

35

Nobody knows exactly when these books were written. Ancient Hindus wrote on banana leaves and birch bark. These materials were fragile, and the original documents did not last long. Some historians believe that Sushruta lived around 1000 B.C. Others say he lived around 100 B.C.

Historians do know that by 326 B.C., when Alexander the Great and his army crossed the Indus River, Indian medicine was already very advanced. Experts believe that Indian medicine developed independently and was not influenced by the medicine of Greece or other contemporary civilizations.

PLASTIC SURGERY

The ancient Hindus lived under a harsh system of laws. Judges punished lawbreakers by ordering that parts of their bodies be cut off or mangled. Thieves might have a hand or an arm amputated. Liars might be burned on the face. To meet the needs of such people, Hindu doctors developed procedures for repairing disfigurement—a technology we now call plastic, or reconstructive, surgery.

Warfare also created a need for plastic surgery. Unlike the ancient Greeks and Romans, Hindu warriors did not wear protective helmets. Many soldiers thus had ears or noses cut off in battle, or suffered other disfiguring facial wounds.

Another reason for plastic surgery in ancient India came from the custom of piercing and stretching earlobes. Parents had their children's earlobes stretched to ward off evil spells and spirits. Physicians pierced earlobes with sharp instruments, then plugged and enlarged the holes with wads of cotton and wood. They also tied lead weights on earlobes to stretch them. Such artificially shaped earlobes were thought to be beautiful.

Not surprisingly, holes in long, dangling earlobes tended to get caught on objects, and earlobes ripped open. Heavy earrings also tore earlobes. Ancient Indian surgeons learned to repair the damage and create a new earlobe. Modern plastic surgeons still use the same procedure on patients who lose earlobes because of cancer, accidents, or other problems. Here is how Sushruta described the technology:

> A surgeon well-versed in the knowledge of surgery should slice off a patch of living flesh from the cheek-ear [the neck right behind the ear] of a person devoid of ear-lobes in a manner so as to have one of its ends attached to the former seat. Then the part, where the artificial ear-lobe is to be made, should be slightly scarified [scratched with a knife] and the living flesh, full of blood and sliced off as previously described, should be adhesioned to it.

One of the most basic procedures in modern plastic surgery is based directly on this ancient surgical technology. It involves cutting an area of skin and underlying tissue in the shape of a long U. The flap of tissue, called a pedicle flap, looks much like a tongue, with one end free and the other attached to the body.

Surgeons lift the free end, then sew it onto a damaged part of the body. First, they scrape, or scarify, the attachment site, as Sushruta advised, so the raw pieces of tissue can grow together. Once the raw surfaces have healed, the surgeons cut and free the base of the flap.

Ancient Indian surgeons even used the pedicle flap technique to create new noses for those who had lost theirs. From the unfortunate person's forehead, the surgeon cut a triangular flap of tissue, shaped much like a kite. The broad end was lifted free from the forehead, and the narrow portion was left attached to the bridge of the nose.

The surgeon then lifted the flap down over the nose opening and stitched it in place. He produced new nostrils by molding the flap around two hollow tubes. The modern operation for nose reconstruction uses the same technique.

ANT SUTURES

Indian surgeons sometimes had to operate on the intestines after people were injured in battle or gored by animals. These operations were especially dangerous. When a surgeon stitched up an incision in the intestines, digested food or fecal material tended to seep out through the needle holes.

The sutures, or stitches, acted like wicks. Just as cotton string can draw water from a glass, early sutures—made of cotton, linen, silk, or other fibers—drew liquid out of the intestines. A single drop of such liquid, smaller than the period at the end of this sentence, contains millions of bacteria. The bacteria caused horrible infections.

Hindu surgeons developed an ingenious solution. Before starting intestinal surgery, they collected large Bengali ants. Some were almost an inch long. These insects will clamp down their powerful jaws to grasp food, enemies, or almost any object they touch.

The surgeons carefully held one ant at the very end of an incision and let it clamp down, drawing the cut edges of the intestine together. They placed another ant alongside. And another. And another, until ant jaws sealed the entire incision. Then the surgeons cut away the ants' bodies, and the jaws stayed firmly clamped in place.

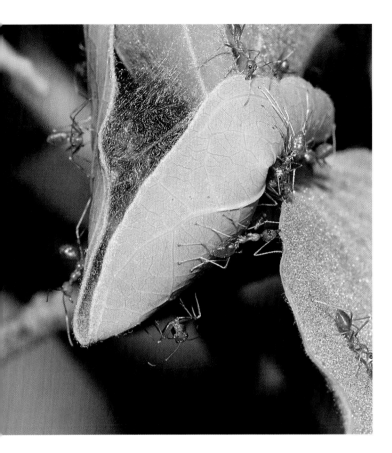

Tailor, or weaver, ants use their strong jaws to make nests out of leaves. People have used this Indian species, *Oecophyla smaragdina,* to close wounds.

Sushruta advised surgeons how to proceed next: "After that the intestines with the heads of the ants attached should be gently pushed back into the [abdominal] cavity and reinstated in their original situation therein."

Surgeons then sewed up layers of muscle and skin in the incision with a needle and ordinary sutures. Within a few weeks, the patient's immune system would attack and destroy the ant jaws, turning them into liquid that the body absorbed. By that time, the intestines were safely healed. The Bengali ants are the forerunner of modern surgical stapling, in which surgeons close intestinal wounds with stainless steel staples.

Spilling Their Guts

Indian surgeons had techniques for treating another messy and dangerous problem with abdominal wounds. Lengths of intestine, sometimes many feet long, often spilled out of wounds and hung outside the body. Left outside, intestines dried out and became infected. Infections caused slow, agonizing death.

For doctors, stuffing the slippery guts back into a wound was difficult. Sushruta suggested several ways of getting the intestines to retract, or slip back inside the abdomen. One of the most effective methods involved making the patient vomit. Vomiting caused the abdominal muscles to contract and literally sucked the guts back inside. Another technique was to have a strong man lift the patient into the air and shake him up and down.

Sushruta recommended that intestines first be washed gently with milk to prevent infection. If the intestines had already dried out, the surgeon was instructed to moisten them with a solution of milk and melted butter.

Teaching Aids

Modern doctors spend a great deal of time practicing surgical and other techniques. They must learn how hard to press down on scalpels and how tightly to pull stitches. They must develop hand-eye coordination and manual dexterity. They practice on cadavers (dead bodies) or animals rather than on living people. Plastic models also help prepare surgeons for treating real patients.

Ancient Hindu physicians also practiced their techniques on models. Student physicians practiced making incisions on watermelons and cucumbers. They stitched up pieces of animal hide to practice suturing human tissue. Young surgeons practiced amputating limbs of dead animals. They practiced lancing abscesses on leather bags filled with mud or water. They practiced cautery (burning wounds to prevent bleeding or infection) on pieces of fresh meat. Since there were no effective anesthetics to relieve pain in ancient times, it was very important for surgeons to perform their tasks quickly.

Indian surgeons had a wide assortment of instruments. The *Sushruta Samhita* lists more than 120 surgical instruments, including scalpels, forceps, probes, saws, needles, and retractors. Forceps took their names from the shape of their jaws. The lion forceps, for instance, had huge jaws for grasping big structures such as bones. The crocodile forceps had long, narrow jaws. Jaws of the hawk forceps were shaped like a scoop. The heron mouth forceps had long, narrow, sharply pointed jaws for removing splinters and other objects deep within wounds. Young surgeons practiced proper use of forceps by picking seeds out of different kinds of fruit.

PUBLIC HEALTH KNOWLEDGE

Ancient Indian physicians knew that patients themselves could do much to stay healthy. Indian doctors urged people to bathe regularly, brush their teeth, exercise, and eat a proper diet. They knew that flies transmit disease by landing on human and animal feces, then on food. So they advised people to avoid fly-infested foods. During

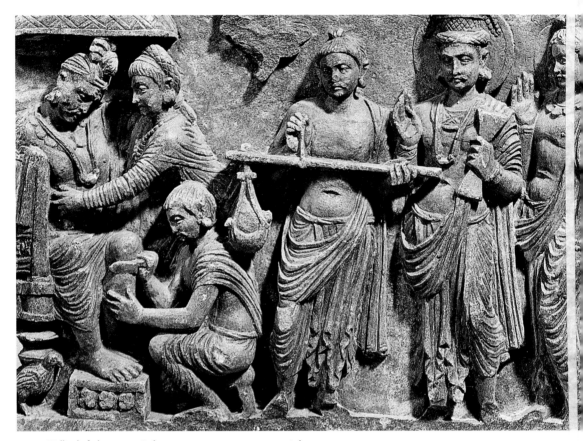

Wall relief showing an Indian surgeon operating on a man's leg

epidemics, widespread outbreaks of disease, doctors advised people to avoid drinking water and eating raw fruits or vegetables—since disease spread through water and raw food contaminated by feces.

SMALLPOX VACCINE

Many times throughout history, epidemics of a highly infectious disease called smallpox have swept through the world. The disease, caused by a virus, has killed hundreds of millions of people and scarred or blinded even more.

Smallpox victims get a rash on the face and other parts of the body. At first the rash looks like thousands of small pimples. Then the pimples become larger and fill with pus. They break open and form crusty scabs that fall off. Each scab leaves a deep, craterlike scar. Smallpox was so common in earlier times that people often stood out in a crowd if their faces were not disfigured by its scars. Fortunately, after getting smallpox once, people develop lifelong immunity, or resistance, to the disease.

In 1796, Edward Jenner, an English physician, developed a vaccine to prevent smallpox. The last naturally occurring cases of smallpox appeared in 1977, and in 1980 the World Health Organization declared that smallpox had been eradicated, or totally eliminated, from the earth.

An ancient Hindu medical technology may have prevented many smallpox cases before Jenner's vaccine appeared. The Indians vaccinated people against smallpox with a technique called variolation. They took dried scabs from smallpox patients and applied them to the skin or inside the noses of healthy people. Sometimes, healthy people ate the scabs. The procedure exposed healthy people to the smallpox virus, so that they too developed lifelong immunity without getting the actual disease.

THE FIRST HOSPITALS

Television programs show that patients receive the very latest in high-tech medical care in hospitals. The idea of bringing sick or injured people to a central facility originated in ancient times.

Some of the first references to hospitals come from ancient India. An inscription carved into a slab of rock around 226 B.C. honored an Indian ruler named Asoka for building hospitals. Other records indicate that hospitals operated in what is now Sri Lanka, an island in the Indian Ocean, around 437 B.C.

We know very little about these hospitals. They may have been only temporary structures. The first permanent hospitals were built by the ancient Romans, several centuries later.

4

ANCIENT CHINA

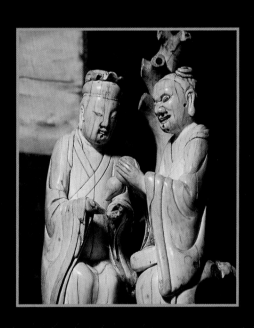

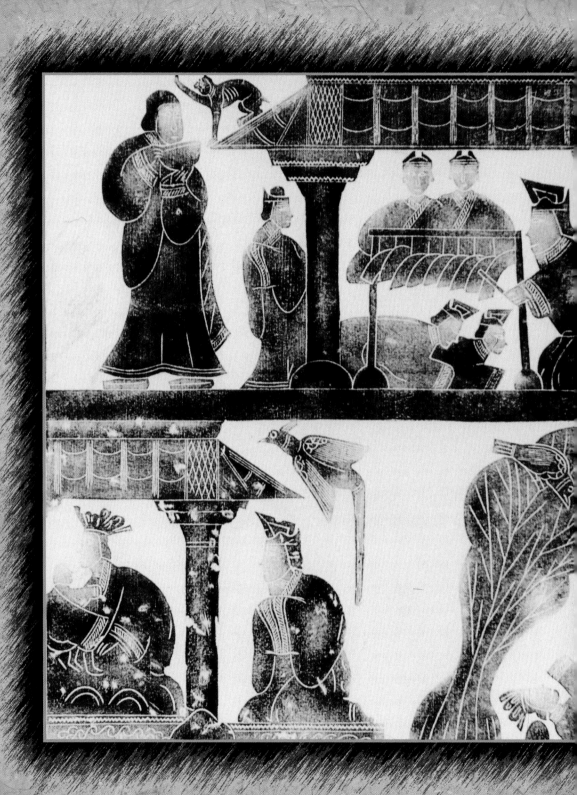

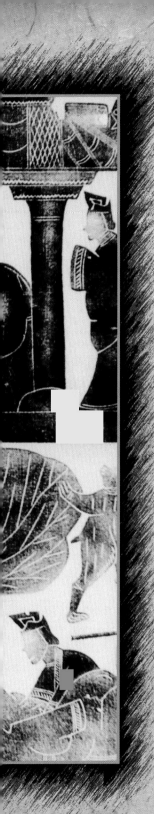

Han dynasty (207 B.C.–A.D. 220) rubbing showing Confucius (top, second from right) lecturing

hinese civilization began between 5000 and 3000 B.C. in the Yellow River Valley in northern China. There, Stone Age people settled into small farming villages that grew into thriving cities. The river provided water for drinking, irrigation, fishing, and transportation. When the river flooded the land, it left behind layers of rich yellow soil that grew abundant crops.

As civilization became more advanced, local kings in northern China established the country's first dynasty, or ruling family. Called the Shang dynasty, it ruled from about 1766 B.C. until about 1122 B.C. The Shang civilization spread to many other areas of China.

Medicine under the Shang involved much magic and superstition, as it did in other early civilizations. Real medical technology emerged after the Chou dynasty conquered the Shang in 1122 B.C. By about 500 B.C., physicians had joined priests and sorcerers in China. Around 500 B.C., the Chinese philosopher Confucius

47

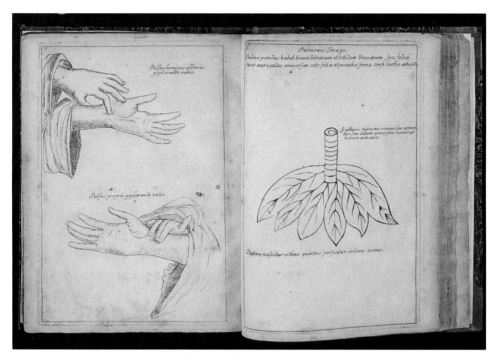

In the fourth century A.D., Wang Shu-ho published a treatise on the pulse. The illustrations show how to take someone else's pulse (top left), and how to take one's own pulse (bottom left).

wrote that a person "without persistence will never make a good magician or a good physician."

Much of our knowledge about ancient Chinese medicine comes from two books. One is the *Chou Li*, or "Institutions of the Chou." It describes government organization under the Chou dynasty. The other is the *Huang Ti Nei Ching* (or *Nei Ching*), which means "The Yellow Emperor's Classic on Internal Medicine." In this book, the Yellow Emperor holds dialogues, or discussions, with his prime minister, Ch'i Po.

The Yellow Emperor is a mysterious figure in Chinese history. Nobody knows exactly when he lived, or whether he was real or legendary. Some Chinese believe that he reigned as early as 2600 B.C. The *Nei Ching* probably was written between 479 and 300 B.C.

HIGH BLOOD PRESSURE

In the 1950s and 1960s, American doctors began to realize that too much salt in the diet can contribute to high blood pressure. High blood pressure, or hypertension, increases the risk of heart attack and stroke, which are the leading causes of death for Americans.

The ancient Chinese were aware of salt's effects thousands of years ago. The *Nei Ching* noted, "If too much salt is used for food, the pulse hardens." A "hardened" pulse, felt in blood vessels in the wrist or neck, means that pressure inside the blood vessels is high.

SPECIALISTS ABOUND

When modern people need medical help, they usually go to a general, or primary care, physician. This doctor can treat most common diseases. She or he also can refer patients to specialists for advanced care.

This approach dates to ancient China. The *Chou Li* tells us that the ruling dynasty had a chief physician. "All the people. . . who suffer from ordinary diseases, head diseases, or wounds, come to him. Thereupon he orders the various physicians to share among them the treatment of these diseases." Other physicians specialized in treating infected ulcers, cuts, or fractures. Some even specialized in allergies and respiratory problems. The *Chou Li* describes physicians who treated "special diseases for each season. In spring there are headaches and troubles with the head. In summer there

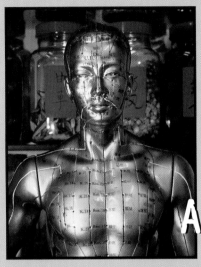

Ancient
Medical
Technology
Rediscovered:

Acupuncture

The Yellow Emperor would have smiled in delight at a 1996 announcement from the U.S. Food and Drug Administration. The FDA had officially approved a "new" medical instrument as safe and effective for use by physicians. The instrument? Acupuncture needles.

The ancient Chinese believed that most diseases resulted from an imbalance between the two life forces, *yin* and *yang*. The forces are supposed to flow in channels, or meridians, that spread out over the body. Fourteen major meridians lead to 361 specific points. Piercing the skin with acupuncture needles is supposed to restore a balance between yin and yang and restore health. Some physicians believe acupuncture can relieve headaches, arthritis, back pain, muscle disorders, and many other diseases.

Western physicians and patients discovered acupuncture in the 1970s after President Richard Nixon visited China. Few Americans had ever visited the country, and Westerners knew little about Chinese medicine. China was then regarded as one of the United States's greatest enemies.

Left: Modern Chinese bronze model of the
Zheng Jiu Toing Ren, or Acupuncture Man

Scientists who accompanied Nixon on the trip brought back amazing stories about acupuncture. They watched Chinese patients undergo major surgery with no anesthetics other than a few acupuncture needles stuck in their skin. Since then, many studies have shown that acupuncture can be effective in treating some diseases.

Acupuncture's origins are lost in history. Some ancient medical texts describe flint acupuncture needles, suggesting that the technique may have originated in the Stone Age. Sets of gold and silver acupuncture needles were discovered in tombs dating to the first century B.C. Archaeologists have also discovered bronze needles, which could be acupuncture needles, that were made in the 900s B.C. Acupuncture as described in the *Nei Ching* was a completely developed system of medicine. It probably began centuries earlier. The *Nei Ching* also describes a related technique, moxibustion, which involves burning small piles of an herb called moxa on the skin. Yes, it does hurt.

Acupuncture is still practiced exactly as it was more than two thousand years ago. Modern practitioners insert and twirl needles and sometimes burn moxa at the same body points mapped out by ancient Chinese physicians. They use the same acupuncture charts and dolls (small human figures) showing point locations. Points may be some distance from ailments they control. Needling a point in the hand, for instance, is a cure for headache. Acupuncture needles are thin and cause little pain.

Until 1996, the FDA classified acupuncture needles as experimental devices. Therefore most health insurance companies would not pay for acupuncture treatment. With that barrier eliminated, acupuncture may become as popular in the twenty-first century as it was in the Yellow Emperor's day.

are ulcers and sores. In autumn there are fevers and colds. In winter there are coughs and troubles of breathing."

A Good Idea Travels West

Modern physicians must take many examinations to test their knowledge and ability. Students must pass an examination before entering medical school. Medical school graduates must pass a test to get a license to practice medicine. Physicians must pass other exams to become specialists. Later in their careers, physicians must take written tests to show that they have kept up to date with new medical advances.

Testing helps protect patients from incompetent physicians. The practice began in ancient China, where the government graded physicians according to their performance. The *Chou Li* describes how the Chinese government made physicians take regular written exams. These were given as early as 165 B.C. and were the first such exams recorded anywhere in the world.

It took 1,300 years for European governments to start offering patients similar assurance. Historians believe that the idea passed slowly from China through the ancient Middle East and reached Sicily in the twelfth century. There, in A.D. 1140, a ruler named Roger II the Norman made the first law requiring physicians to take formal written examinations.

ANCIENT GREECE

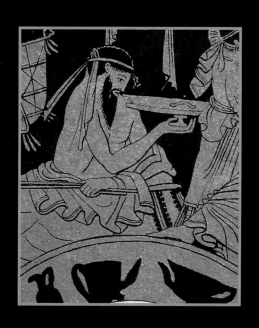

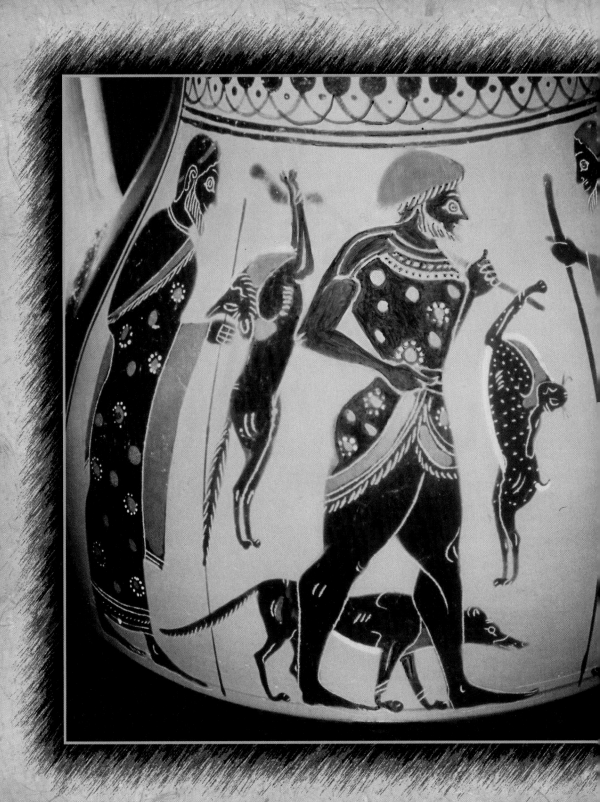

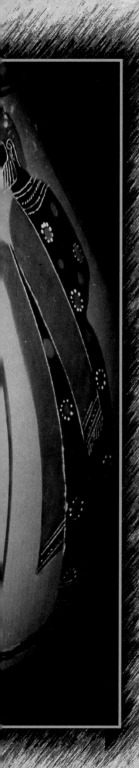

Greek hunter and his dog, painted around
550 B.C.

The first Greek civilization began around 1650 B.C., when warrior-kings built palaces at Thebes, Mycenae, and other locations in southern Greece. Historians call this the Mycenaean civilization, because Mycenae was the most important town.

The early Greeks were influenced by a still earlier civilization on Crete, an island a few hundred miles away in the Mediterranean Sea. This was the Minoan civilization, which began around 2600 B.C. and was named after a legendary king, Minos.

The greatest period of Greek civilization began about 800 B.C. Called the Hellenic Age, it included the birth of democracy in Athens and the lifetimes of famous philosophers, writers, and artists. Many of Greece's contributions to medical technology occurred during this period.

Between 431 and 404 B.C., a great war between the city-states of Athens and Sparta weakened ancient Greece. In 338 B.C., Philip of

Macedonia conquered the Greek city-states. His son, Alexander the Great, then conquered much of the Mediterranean and Near Eastern world, from Egypt to India. Medical technology flowed into Greece from the conquered lands. In Egypt, Alexander founded the city of Alexandria, which became the center for Greek medicine. Alexander died in 323 B.C., marking the start of the Hellenistic Age.

MEDICINE'S SYMBOL

Like the ancient Egyptians, the Greeks had a god of health, Asclepius. Asclepius probably was a living person who was elevated to the status of a god after death. Homer mentions Asclepius in *The Iliad*, a poem about the Greek siege of Troy that took place from 1194 to 1184 B.C.

Asclepius believed that snakes and serpents were sacred. He adopted serpents coiled around a staff as his symbol. The modern medical profession uses a similar symbol, called the caduceus, or the staff of Hermes (or Mercury). It consists of two snakes coiled around a staff with a pair of wings on top.

The Greeks built temples in honor of Asclepius that functioned like modern health clinics or spas. Sick people went to the temples to be cured. The temples were built near mineral springs, in dry, sunny places where the climate was supposed to be especially healthful. Priests trained in medicine staffed the temples. They treated patients with special diets, mineral baths, massage, medicines, and other procedures. The temples also served as medical schools.

Archaeologists have found and restored the remains of many of these temples to Asclepius. Two of the most

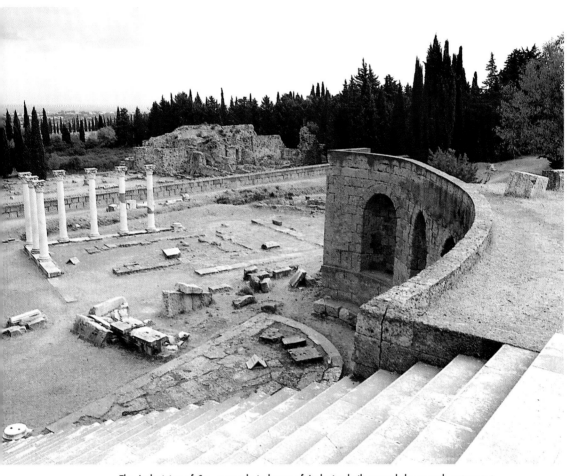

The Asclepieion of Cos, a temple in honor of Asclepius built around the second century B.C.

famous were located on the island of Cos and in the city of Pergamos.

Some historians believe that the Greeks borrowed the idea of a god of health from Egypt's famous physician-god, Imhotep. Greece established trading colonies in Egypt in the seventh century B.C. Seeing that Egyptian medicine was superior to their own, the colonists embraced Egypt's medical technology and brought it back home.

FATHER OF MEDICINE

Hippocrates was a Greek physician who made medicine a profession and ended some of the age-old connections between medicine and religion. He discarded the idea that angry gods punished people with disease, and he developed a scientific approach to treating patients. Hippocrates taught physicians to carefully observe each patient's symptoms and to select an appropriate treatment.

Hippocrates was born around 460 B.C. on the island of Cos and lived long—between 85 and 109 years. While teaching at the great medical school on Cos, Hippocrates, and perhaps his students, wrote a summary of Greek medicine. It included the books *Epidemics*, *Prognostics*, *Ancient Medicine*, and *Airs, Waters and Places*. Physicians used these books for almost two thousand years. Modern physicians call these writings the Hippocratic Collection.

Many modern people strive for a "healthy lifestyle." They try to eat a low-fat diet, get regular exercise, and avoid dangerous practices such as smoking. Hippocrates may have been the "father" of the healthy lifestyle. He urged people to eat a good diet and to get regular exercise. But some of his dietary advice was bad. For example, Hippocrates thought that fresh fruits and vegetables were unhealthy. But his recommendation about the best exercise for inactive people—walking—is still given by modern doctors.

Of all Hippocrates' contributions, the use of case histories is the most important. Case histories consist of carefully arranged descriptions of patients, symptoms, diagnoses,

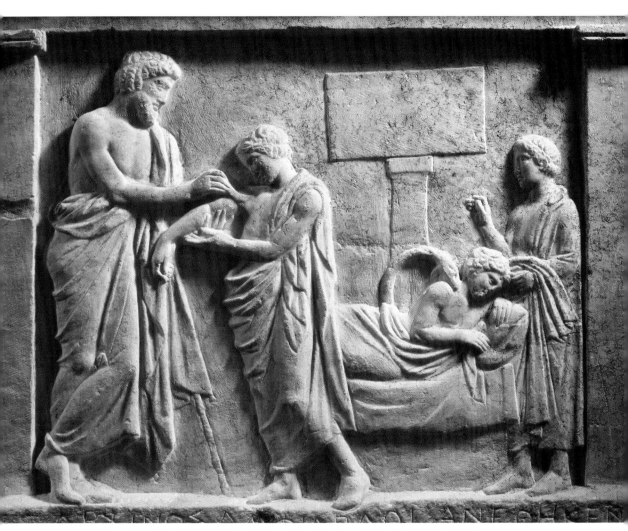

Relief from the sanctuary of Oropos, dedicated to the physician Amphiarios, showing Hippocrates treating a patient

treatments, and outcomes. Modern physicians use Hippocrates' approach in medical record keeping, teaching, and reporting. One case history began:

Silenus lived on the Broad-way, near the house of Evalcidas. From fatigue, drinking, and unseasonable exercises, he was seized with fever. He began with having pain in the loins; he had heaviness of the head and there was stiffness of the neck. On the first day the alvine [stomach or intestinal] discharges were bilious [from the liver], unmixed, frothy, highly colored, and copious [plentiful]; urine black, have a black sediment; he was thirsty, tongue dry; no sleep at night. On the second, acute fever; stools, more copious, thinner, frothy; urine black; an discomfortable night; slight delirium.

Another said:

Philiscus, who lived by the wall, took to bed on the first day of acute fever; he sweated; towards night was uneasy. On the second day all symptoms were exacerbated [worsened]; late in the evening had a proper stool [bowel movement] from a small clyster [enema], the night quiet. On the third day, early in the morning and until noon he appeared to be free from fever; towards evening, acute fever, with sweating, thirst, tongue parched; passed black urine; night uncomfortable, no sleep; he was delirious on all subjects.

AN ETHICAL CODE FOR DOCTORS

Hippocrates made his students take a pledge, called the Hippocratic Oath. For almost 2,500 years, the oath has served as a code of conduct for the medical profession. It has helped physicians decide what to do and not do when dealing with patients. Thousands of new doctors have taken the Hippocratic Oath over the centuries, raising a hand and swearing to adhere to its principles.

Ideas about ethical behavior change over the years.

Doctors and the rest of society no longer accept some parts of the Hippocratic Oath. In Hippocrates' time, for instance, no respectable physician would perform surgery, which was regarded by the Greeks as a craft, rather than an art like medicine. The oath thus forbade using "the knife."

American doctors in modern times follow a code of medical ethics published by the American Medical Association. Yet the Hippocratic Oath remains the most famous guide for judging what is right and wrong in the relationship between doctors and patients. Most medical schools use variations of the oath at graduation ceremonies. You've probably heard some of its words:

> I swear by Apollo Physician, by Asclepius, by Health, by Panacea and by all the gods and goddesses, making them my witness that I will carry out, according to my ability and judgment, this oath and this indenture....I will use treatment to help the sick according to my ability and judgment, but never with a view to injury and wrongdoing. Neither will I administer a poison to anybody when asked to do so nor will I suggest such a course. Similarly I will not give a woman a pessary to cause abortion. But I will keep pure and holy both my life and my art. I will not use the knife, not even, verily, on sufferers from [kidney] stone, but will give place to such as are craftsmen therein. Into whatsoever houses I enter, I will enter to help the sick, and I will abstain from all intentional wrongdoing and harm, especially from abusing the bodies of man or woman, bond or free. And whatsoever I shall see or hear in the course of my profession, as well as outside my profession in my intercourse with men, if it be what should not be published abroad, I will never divulge, holding such things to be secrets. Now if I carry out this oath, and break it not, may I gain for ever reputation among all men for my life and for my art; but if I transgress it and forswear myself, may the opposite befall me.

"To Cut Up"

Our modern medical term *anatomy* comes from Greek words that mean "to cut up." The study of human anatomy involves cutting up, or dissecting, bodies. Anatomy is one of the first courses medical students must take. Doctors must know how the body is put together in order to diagnose and treat diseases.

The ancient Greeks laid the basis for this critical area of medical science. Alcmaeon of Croton, who lived around 500 B.C., performed dissections. He wrote a description of the optic nerve in the eye and the Eustachian tube inside the ear. Two other pioneers of anatomy were the Greek physician Herophilus of Chaludon and his student, Erasistratus.

Herophilus started a school of anatomy at Alexandria. Some historians think he was the first physician to dissect the human body. He wrote the first detailed description of the brain and recognized the brain as the seat of intelligence. He described differences between two key parts of the brain, the cerebrum and cerebellum, and suggested that nerves are involved in the senses. He also recognized the difference between arteries, which carry fresh, oxygen-rich blood away from the heart, and veins, which carry blood from body tissues back to the heart.

The philosopher Aristotle (384–322 B.C.) also advanced the study of anatomy. He studied plants and animals and originated a field of biomedical science called comparative anatomy. Researchers in this field compare the bodies of different kinds of animals and place animals in biological categories. Aristotle dissected animals and taught physicians that their theories about disease should be based on facts—things that can be observed.

Ancient Human Experimentation

Modern medical researchers sometimes conduct experiments on living people. They use volunteer subjects to test new drugs, instruments, and other technology. Such experiments are often the only way to determine if a technology is safe and effective. Committees of experts review the experiments before allowing them to proceed. They make sure the experiments are ethical and that all participation is voluntary.

Herophilus and Erasistratus performed what may be the first medical experiments on humans. These were much different from experiments performed in modern times. The Roman physician Cornelius Celsus gave a gruesome account:

> Herophilus and Erasistratus...laid open men whilst alive—criminals received out of prison from the kinds—and whilst these were still breathing, observed parts of which beforehand nature had concealed, their position, color, shape, size, arrangement, hardness, softness, smoothness, relation, processes and depressions of each, and whether any part is inserted into or received into another.

Celsus condemned the experiments as "dire cruelty." Physicians, he said, could get the same knowledge by observing organs exposed by wounds in gladiators (professional warriors) and accident victims.

The First Shrink

Asclepiades of Bithynia was born around 124 B.C. He introduced a number of principles for treating people with mental illness that are the basis for modern psychiatry. He

A Plague of Hiccups

The Great Plague of Athens struck Greece between 430 and 425 B.C. Some historians believe it killed one-third to one-half of Greece's population—up to three hundred thousand people. The plague helped to end the Hellenic Age of Greece.

In his book *The History of the Peloponnesian War,* the historian Thucydides described the plague as a terrible disease. Victims suddenly got high fevers and sore throats. Blisters broke out on their skin, they vomited green material, had diarrhea, and suffered from such intense thirst that they couldn't drink enough water. "The bodies of dying men lay one upon the other," Thucydides wrote, "and half-dead creatures reeled about the streets and gathered all round the fountains in their longing for water." Some developed hiccups that would not stop. At the same time, the plague struck other parts of the world, including Rome, which then was only a small town.

What caused the epidemic? Influenza? A bad form of measles? Bubonic plague? Scientists have argued over these and other possibilities. After 2,400 years, scientists think they have an answer.

Experts believe that the plague of Athens was an epidemic of Ebola virus. Ebola caused worldwide alarm in 1995 when it killed 242 people in Kikwit, Zaire, in Africa. The disease was the topic of a popular motion picture, *Outbreak.* Scientists say there are many similarities between Ebola and the symptoms reported by Thucydides.

One strong argument: hiccups. Ebola is the only known infectious disease that causes severe hiccuping in many of its victims. Another: African green monkeys transmit the Ebola virus to humans. Not far from modern Athens, archaeologists have found ancient wall paintings depicting African green monkeys. Greek traders apparently brought the monkeys back from voyages to Africa. Ebola thus may not be the new, or emerging, disease that scientists first thought.

People still fear diseases that caused great suffering in ancient times. Modern medical professionals still struggle to cope with diseases that occurred long before Hippocrates' birth. Cancer. Heart attacks. Arthritis. Diabetes. Tooth decay. Gum disease. Ebola virus may be another dramatic addition to the list.

An African green monkey, *Cercopithecus aethiops*

urged that mentally ill people be treated humanely. He introduced occupational therapy, exercises to help patients with memory problems, and music therapy to calm anxious patients.

Before Asclepiades, mentally ill patients were kept in dark rooms. Physicians thought darkness had a soothing effect. Asclepiades realized that some mentally ill people had more hallucinations in the dark, and he moved them into well-lit rooms. Many of his ideas were lost and not used again until the early twentieth century.

THE PUS PULLER

Few medical devices are more important than the hypodermic syringe. Doctors and nurses use millions of syringes each year to give injections of medicine, take samples of blood, and drain fluid from the body.

Nobody knows for certain who made the first syringe. The first description of a syringe appears in a book written by Hero of Alexandria. In the first century A.D., he described a syringe consisting of a piston inside a hollow cylinder, open at one end. When the piston was pushed, air or liquid inside the cylinder squirted out the end. The cylinder-and-piston syringe was invented around 280 B.C. by Ktesibios, an engineer who also lived in Alexandria. But syringes may have been in use long before that time.

The ancient Greeks used syringes mostly to suck pus out of pimples, boils, and infected wounds. The Greek name for the syringe, *pyulkos*, and the Latin name, *pyulcus*, mean "pus puller." Beginning in the mid-nineteenth century, physicians began to use syringes to inject medicines directly into veins, tissue, and muscle.

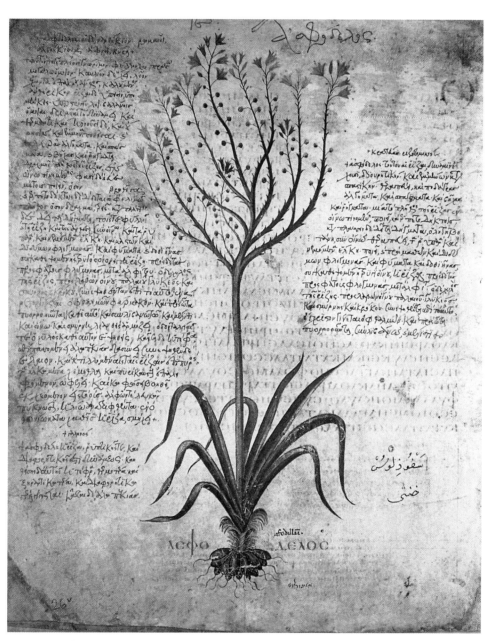

A page from *De Materia Medica,* a book written in the first century A.D. that describes the medicinal properties of hundreds of different plants

MEDICINAL PLANTS

Pedanius Dioscorides, a Greek physician who lived in the first century A.D., wrote one of the most complete descriptions of ancient medicinal plants. His book, *De Materia Medica*, described five hundred medicinal plants and carried illustrations of many of them. It was the most respected book on drugs in the world for almost 1,200 years.

6

ANCIENT ROME

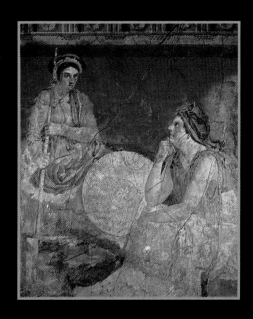

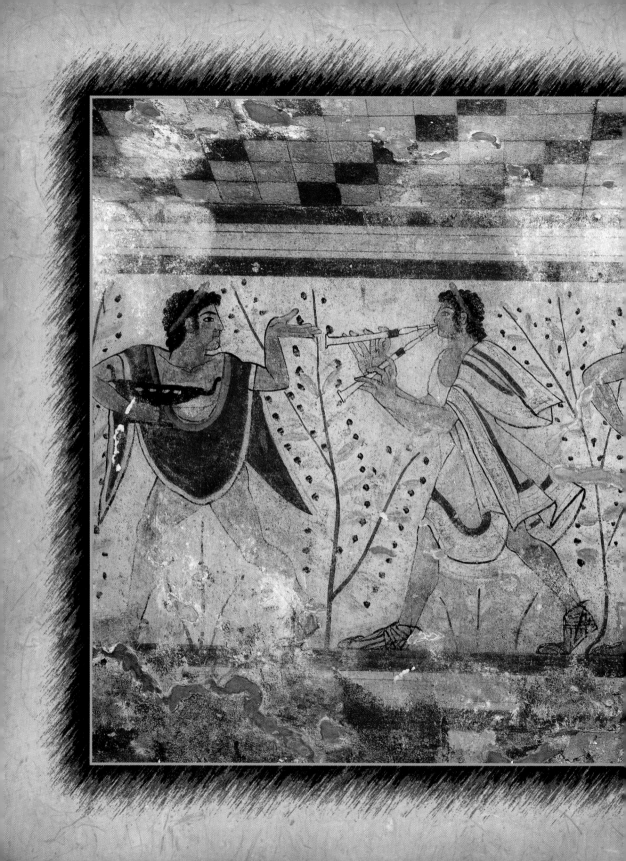

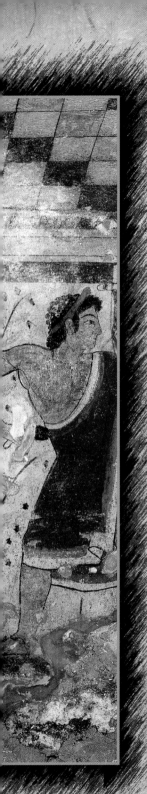

Painting of an offering-bearer and musicians from the Tomb of the Leopards in Tarquinia, Italy

A group of nomadic people called the Latins grazed herds of sheep in central Italy below the Tiber River from 2000 B.C. until 750 B.C. Then they settled into permanent farming villages that eventually grew into the city of Rome. It was built on seven hills along the Tiber.

The Latins were only one of several groups living in Italy. The Etruscans lived to the north and west. The Greeks had established city-states throughout southern Italy and in Sicily. In 509 B.C., the Latins overthrew the Etruscans, who had ruled them for a hundred years, and established a republic. The republic lasted for five hundred years, as Rome conquered many other countries and grew into the greatest ancient civilization.

For hundreds of years, the Romans had no physicians, surgeons, or other formal medical care. Why not? Pliny the Elder, the great Roman historian who lived from A.D. 23 to 79, concluded that the ancient Romans were too cheap. Pliny wrote of the early Romans' dislike of physicians: "It was not medicine itself that the ancient condemned, but medicine as a profession, mainly because they refused to pay fees to profiteers in order to save their own lives." Romans also considered medicine a low-class occupation, fit only for foreigners or slaves.

The Romans conquered other countries and adopted foreign technologies and ways of life. These naturally included medical technologies that offered people much better treatment than old Roman folk remedies. Rome borrowed much of its medical technology from the Greeks. Greek medicine was so advanced that Rome, in the words of one ancient writer, was "swept along on the puffs of the clever brains of Greece."

Experts think that the Romans also adopted Indian medical technology. There are many indications that the two civilizations traded with each other. The Romans loved

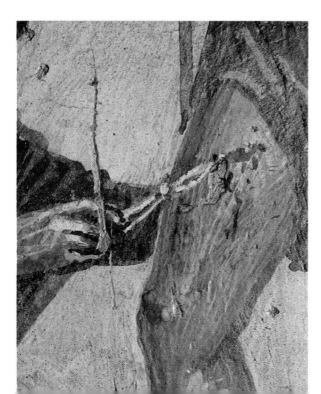

Detail of a painting from the Casa di Sirico in Pompeii, Italy, showing a surgeon stitching a wound

pepper on their food and imported it from India. Traders also brought back Indian drugs and surgical procedures. One Roman historian complained that people ignored medicinal plants growing around their own country because so many effective drugs came from India.

In the third century B.C., Alexandria was the medical and scientific capital of the world. It had a great medical library and great physicians. As Greek civilization declined around 220 B.C., famous Greek physicians began to leave Alexandria and other cities to live in the new rising empire of Rome. Thus most of Rome's best physicians were Greek.

THE WORLD'S MOST FAMOUS MEDICAL TEXTBOOK

Cornelius Celsus was a Roman nobleman who owned great expanses of land. He lived during the reign of Tiberius, emperor from A.D. 14 to 37. Around A.D. 30, Celsus wrote *De Medicina*—"On Medicine." It was the medical section of Celsus's much longer book on warfare, farming, and many other topics. *De Medicina* consisted of eight sections that described treatments for disease, special diets, surgical operations, and other wonders more advanced than anything then available.

After Rome fell in the fifth century A.D., the Dark Ages began in Europe. Many achievements of ancient Greece and Rome were lost. When the Dark Ages ended and the Renaissance, or rebirth of learning, began around 1350, Italian scholars discovered a five-hundred-year-old copy of *De Medicina*. The printing press was invented in 1455, and in 1478 *De Medicina* became the first medical book to be printed. It was used by physicians throughout the world until the middle of the eighteenth century.

CELSIAN LEGACIES TO MODERN MEDICINE

Doctors around the world still use Celsus's definition of inflammation. Inflammation is a reaction to disease or injury. It can result from infections; surgery; accidents; cancer; exposure to extreme heat, cold, chemicals, or radiation; and autoimmune diseases, in which the immune system mistakenly attacks and destroys body tissue. Celsus realized that there are four basic signs of inflammation, which he stated in Latin as, "rubor et tumor cum calore et dolore." No physician has ever provided a more precise definition of the symptoms of inflammation: "redness and swelling with heat and pain."

Modern doctors recognize two basic kinds of disease: chronic and acute. Chronic diseases, such as arthritis, last a long time. Patients may live with them for decades. In contrast, acute diseases, such as infections, end quickly. The end may be good or bad. The patient may recover quickly or die quickly. Celsus left modern medicine with a beautifully precise definition of acute: "Cito vel tollunt hominem, vel ipsi cito finiuntur." Acute diseases "either finish the man quickly, or finish themselves quickly."

"TO CUT UP," CONTINUED . . .

Ancient anatomy that began with Herophilus in Greece reached a peak with Claudius Galen in Rome. Born in Pergamos in A.D. 129, Galen studied medicine in Alexandria. He learned a great deal about wounds and the insides of the human body by treating gladiators in Pergamos.

In A.D. 162, Galen moved to Rome, then capital of the Western world. There, he became physician to Emperor Marcus Aurelius. He learned more about the body by dissecting monkeys and other animals and by studying human skeletons. Galen wrote hundreds of essays that influenced medicine for centuries. He was called "the Prince of Physicians."

One of Galen's most important anatomical discoveries was that a nerve—the recurrent laryngeal nerve—controls speech. Galen operated on a pig to determine if a nerve in the animal's neck controlled breathing. He cut the nerve, and the pig was unable to squeal. The experiment, although harmful to the pig, helped human patients. Physicians then knew to avoid cutting the nerve when operating on humans to remove goiters (enlarged thyroid glands). If the nerve were accidentally cut, patients sometimes could not speak afterward. The recurrent laryngeal nerve is still called Galen's nerve.

Galen put all his knowledge into a 16-volume book, *On Anatomical Procedure*. It is considered to be the first textbook on human anatomy. Galen's book represented the peak of anatomy as a science for 1,500 years. Research on human anatomy stood still until A.D. 1316, when an Italian, Mondino dei Liuzzi—known as the "Restorer of Anatomy"—wrote a famous book on the topic.

TAKING YOUR PULSE

Galen developed one of the most widely used medical tests: taking the pulse. The pulse is the rhythmic expansion and contraction of an artery that can be felt through the skin. Doctors often feel the pulse in a patient's wrist. It mirrors the pumping action of the heart. If the pulse is too fast, too slow, or irregular, it may indicate some form of heart disease.

Around A.D. 170, Galen made the first known use of the pulse to diagnose a patient. In an essay, "On the Pulse," he wrote:

> The heart and all the arteries pulsate with the same rhythm, so that from one you can judge of all. But you could not find any arteries more convenient or more suitable for taking the pulse than those in the wrists, for they are easily visible, as there is little flesh over them, and it is not necessary to strip away any part of the body of clothing for them, as is necessary with many others, and they run in a straight course; and this is of no small help in the accuracy of diagnosis.

Galen described more than five hundred medicines derived from plants. He often mixed these medicines together in complicated prescriptions. Some mixtures contained dozens of ingredients. Modern physicians often describe drugs of natural origin as galenical preparations, after Galen.

THE CESAREAN SECTION

A cesarean section is delivery of a baby through a surgical incision in the mother's abdomen and uterus. Most people falsely believe that the term *cesarean* originated from the surgical birth of Julius Caesar, the Roman emperor who ruled from 48 to 44 B.C.

But experts think that Caesar probably was not born by cesarean section. At the time, the operation was performed only when the mother was dying or dead. Roman law decreed that the operation must be done under those circumstances to increase the empire's population. But Julius Caesar's mother, Aurelia, was alive long after his birth. The name *cesarean* actually may have originated from another

Latin word, *caedare*—"to cut open."

Cesarean sections may have been performed in other civilizations long before Roman times. Surgical births are mentioned in ancient Hindu and Egyptian writings, for instance. One ancient Chinese picture shows the operation being done on a living woman.

ANCIENT EYE SURGERY

Mention eye surgery and people usually think of delicate operations requiring specialists and the most modern, high-tech equipment. Yet ancient surgeons performed cataract surgery—an operation to remove a clouded lens from the eye—at least 2,100 years ago. Hindu surgeons probably invented cataract surgery. But the operation became routine in Roman times.

Sushruta, the ancient Hindu surgeon, wrote a long description in his book of the technique for removing cataracts. Celsus described a technique so similar to Sushruta's that experts believe the Romans may have learned the technology from Indian physicians or books. The ancient technique later became known as couching (from the French word *coucher* meaning "to lay down"). Couching remained the best-known treatment for cataracts until early in the twentieth century.

Modern cataract treatment involves removing the clouded lens from the eye and replacing it with an artificial lens, a contact lens, or strong eyeglasses. Ancient surgeons used a fine needle to carefully push the clouded lens out of the way, into the bottom of the eyeball. Celsus knew the danger of this procedure. If the needle slipped and touched the retina, the tissue-thin membrane at the back of the eye, the patient would go blind. So he advised that the patient be tied down or held still by a strong assistant.

Celsus said the cataract needle should be:

> ...inserted at a spot between the pupil of the eye and the angle adjacent to the temple, away from the middle of the cataract, in such a way that no vein is wounded. When the spot is reached, the needle is to be sloped against the lens itself and rotated gently, guiding it little by little below the pupil. When the cataract has passed below the pupil, it is pressed upon more firmly in order that it may settle below. After this the needle is drawn straight out; and soft wool soaked in white of egg is to be put on, and above this something to check inflammation; and then a bandage.

Ancient people did not have eyeglasses. So a patient's vision would have been badly blurred after cataract surgery. The results, however, must have been far better than vision with the cataract. Experts say that patients with severe nearsightedness may even have had much better vision after surgery. The procedure sometimes changed the shape of the eyeball so that light focused more effectively on the retina.

SURGICAL INSTRUMENTS

Archaeologists have unearthed hundreds of ancient Roman surgical instruments. These instruments were better than most available during the Renaissance—1,200 years later. Some instruments were made with such great precision that surgeons could still use them.

The Roman surgeon's forceps, for example, had jaws that aligned precisely and closed tightly when grasping tissue. A gynecologist's speculum had a high-precision screw mecha-

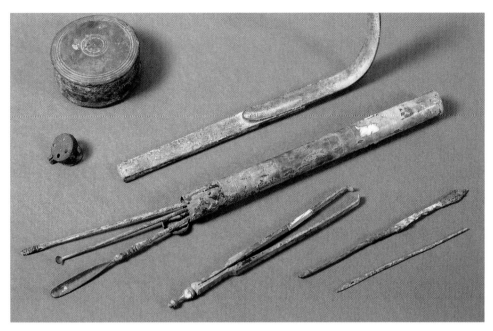

A variety of ancient Roman surgical instruments, including a portable medical kit

nism that gently spread four prongs. Physicians used the instrument to open a woman's vagina when diagnosing and treating certain conditions.

Many surgical instruments were found in the remains of Pompeii, a city that was destroyed when Mount Vesuvius, a volcano, erupted in A.D. 79. Preserved in the volcanic ash were Roman medical kits. These consisted of hollow, pocket-sized metal cylinders with probes, scalpels, and other tools inside.

Celsus described an ingenious device for extracting barbed arrowheads and spearheads from patients. These objects were difficult to remove. Pulling them out usually caused more damage, since the barbs caught on tissue and tore it. Roman doctors used a spoonlike instrument shaped like a modern shoehorn. They inserted the device behind an arrow or spearhead and caught the point in a hole in the end of the spoon. The spoon formed a shield around the barb, which was then removed without causing further damage.

GODDESS OF THE SEWERS

Many of Rome's most important advances in medical technology did not involve the treatment of disease. They involved disease prevention through public health measures. One of the most important measures was sewage disposal.

Every street in Rome had a sewer running along its length. The homes of wealthy people had indoor latrines with pipes that carried waste directly into the sewers. Poorer people used commodes and chamber pots that they emptied into the sewers themselves. There were even pub-

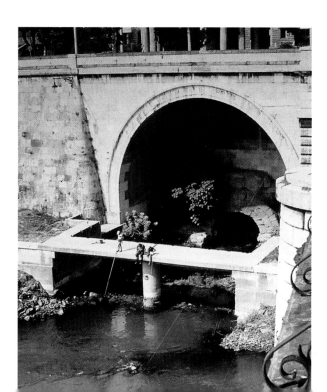

The Cloaca Maxima entering the Tiber River

lic restrooms located along the sewers for use by people away from home.

Water flowed continuously through each sewer, emptying into larger and larger channels. Eventually, all sewers emptied into the Cloaca Maxima—"Big Sewer"—the oldest and most famous sewer in the world. The Cloaca Maxima emptied into the Tiber River.

Construction of Rome's sewer system is thought to have begun during the reign of Tarquinius Priscus, who ruled from 616 to 578 B.C. Engineers and physicians who served as public health officers made sure the sewers worked properly. The Romans considered sanitation to be so important that they even had a goddess who reigned over all the sewers and drains. She was the goddess Cloacina, called "Sweet Cloacina" by many ancient Romans.

Roman sewers were better than many that existed thousands of years later. In many European and American cities, even in the early 1900s, there were no sewers. People simply threw buckets of urine and feces into the streets.

PURE WATER

Another ancient Roman public health advance was delivery of a pure water supply. With sewage emptying into the Tiber River and polluting it, thousands of people got sick from drinking river water.

The republic responded by building its famous aqueduct system, one of the greatest engineering marvels of the ancient world. Aqueducts carried pure water from the countryside into Rome. Appius Claudius built the first aqueduct in 312 B.C. It was 11 miles long and ran almost entirely underground. Other aqueducts were elevated.

Eventually, Rome's population was supplied by at least 11 aqueducts, which brought almost a quarter billion gallons of water into the city each day.

Once again, it was thousands of years before the modern world caught up with ancient technology. Epidemics of cholera and other diseases spread by sewage-contaminated drinking water raged in London, Paris, New York, and other cities into the early 1900s. Thousands of people in developing countries still die each year because they don't have a pure water supply. Romans who lived under Julius Caesar would be shocked, indeed, at the public health conditions that exist in parts of the modern world.

PLASTIC SURGERY

We don't know whether the ancient Romans learned plastic surgery from the pioneer surgeons of the ancient world, the Hindus. But Roman surgeons did perform an operation for repairing a hole in the earlobe caused by wearing heavy earrings.

Celsus's medical textbook describes other simple cosmetic operations, including one for removing brands burned into the skin of slaves. Slaves in ancient Rome occasionally were able to earn their freedom, and they wanted to get rid of their brands so they might look like free people.

THE HOSPITAL SYSTEM

With Roman legions fighting far from home, it was impossible to send wounded soldiers back to Rome for treatment. The Roman military thus developed a new approach. It placed sick and wounded soldiers in special buildings called *valetudinaria*. They were the first permanent hospitals.

Archaeologists have discovered the ruins of at least 25 valetudinaria, spread throughout the old Roman Empire, from modern Scotland to Hungary. Most were built during the second and third centuries A.D., from a standard plan. Small wards opened off a central corridor. Each ward usually held four patients, and each usually had a work area where the staff prepared medicines and food.

Archaeologists have found the remains of medicines and medical instruments in the ruins of some hospitals. In one, archaeologists found seeds of *Hyoscyamus niger,* the henbane plant. It contains the drug scopolamine, which doctors still use to medicate patients prior to surgery. Scopolamine makes people drowsy and erases memory of an operation. Roman physicians combined scopolamine with opium from the opium poppy to produce an effective pain reliever and sedative.

AND AFTERWARD

After the Roman Empire fell in A.D. 476, the clock of medical progress ran backward. Barbarians invaded Rome from the north, and the Dark Ages began. Medicine as a science ceased to exist. Great medical schools and libraries were destroyed. Many manuscripts describing medical technology that had taken centuries to develop were lost.

Monks preserved some manuscripts in monasteries. Other documents were rediscovered centuries later and helped to speed the revival of modern medicine. But for centuries after the end of ancient times, medicine returned to its prehistoric roots in mystery and magic.

Glossary

abscess — a collection of pus inside the body, usually caused by a bacterial infection

anesthetic — a medicine that reduces or eliminates the sensation of pain

antibiotic — a medicine such as penicillin that kills or slows the growth of bacteria and is used to treat bacterial infections

circumcision — surgical removal of the foreskin, a fold of skin that partially covers the end of the penis. It is usually done for cultural or health reasons.

contraception — a device, medicine, or technique to prevent pregnancy

dissection — cutting apart an animal or a plant to study its structure

epidemic — an outbreak of infectious disease that affects a large number of people in the same region at the same time

forceps — small, tongs-like tools used by physicians and dentists for grasping or holding parts of the body

gynecology — the branch of medicine that deals with functions and diseases of the female reproductive system

incision — a cut made into the body to treat a disease

infectious disease — a disease, usually caused by a bacteria or virus, that can be spread from one person to another

plastic surgery — repairing or replacing deformed, damaged, or lost body parts to improve their appearance or function; also called reconstructive surgery

public health — the general health of a community, and steps such as vaccination and sanitation that are taken to maintain and improve it

technology — knowledge applied to satisfy humans' needs and to make life easier, happier, and longer. Technology might consist of instruments, tools, and equipment or of ideas and procedures.

trepanation — a surgical operation in which a circular piece of bone is cut from the skull to expose the brain

BIBLIOGRAPHY

Ackerknecht, Erwin H. *A Short History of Medicine.* Baltimore: The Johns Hopkins University Press, 1982.

Adkins, Lesley, and Roy A. Adkins. *Handbook to Life in Ancient Rome.* New York: Facts on File, 1994.

Clendening, Logan, ed. *Source Book of Medical History.* New York: Dover Publications, Inc., 1942.

Dowling, Harry F. *Medicines for Man.* New York: Alfred A. Knopf, 1970.

Estes, J. Worth. *The Medical Skills of Ancient Egypt.* New York: Science History Publications/USA, 1989.

Garrison, Fielding H. *An Introduction to the History of Medicine.* Springfield, Illinois: Charles C. Thomas, 1954.

James, Peter, and Nick Thorpe. *Ancient Inventions.* New York: Ballantine Books, 1994.

Majno, Guido. *The Healing Hand: Man and Wound in the Ancient World.* Cambridge, Massachusetts: Harvard University Press, 1991.

Nunn, John F. *Ancient Egyptian Medicine.* Norman, Oklahoma: University of Oklahoma Press, 1995.

Saggs, H. W. F. *Civilization Before Greece and Rome.* New Haven: Yale University Press, 1989.

Salzberg, Hugh W. *From Caveman to Chemist.* Washington, DC: American Chemical Society Press, 1991.

Sigerist, Henry E. *A History of Medicine. Vol. 1, Primitive and Archaic Medicine.* New York: Oxford University Press, 1987.

Starr, Chester G., ed. *A History of the Ancient World.* New York: Oxford University Press, 1991.

Trager, James. *The People's Chronology: A Year-by-Year Record of Human Events from Prehistory to the Present.* New York: Holt, Rhinehart and Winston, 1979.

Wain, Harry. *A History of Preventive Medicine.* Springfield, Illinois: Charles C. Thomas, 1974.

Index

acupuncture, 50–51
Alcmaeon of Croton, 62
anatomy, study of, 62, 74–75
ants used as sutures, 38–40
aqueducts, 81–82
Aristotle, 62
Asclepiades of Bithynia, 63–64
Asclepius, 56–57

Broca, Paul, 13

caduceus, as medical symbol, 56
case histories, use of, 58–60
cesarean section, 76–77
Charaka, 35
China: acupuncture, 50–51; blood pressure, 49; pulse, taking of, 48; specialists, medical, 49, 52; writings, medical, 48–49, 51, 52; written examinations for physicians, 52
Claudius Galen, 74–76
Cornelius Celsus, 63, 73–74, 77–78

dentistry, 26, 29–31
doctors. *See* physicians and surgeons
drugs. *See* medications

Ebola virus, 66–67
Egypt: dentistry, 26, 29–31; Hesy Re, 25–26; Imhotep, 24–25; Kom Ombo relief, 28, 29; medications, 27–28, 31–32; Peseshet, 27; specialists, medical, 26–27; surgery, 28; women

as physicians, 27; writings, medical, 23–24, 31, 32
Erasistratus, 62, 63
ethics, medical, 60–61, 63

Great Plague of Athens, 66–67
Greece: Alcmaeon of Croton, 62; anatomy, study of, 62; Asclepiades of Bithynia, 63–64; Asclepius, 56–57; case histories, 58–60; Cornelius Celsus, 63; Ebola virus, 66–67; Erasistratus, 62, 63; experimentation on humans, 63; Great Plague of Athens, 66–67; Herophilus of Chaludon, 62, 63; Hippocrates, 58–61; Hippocratic Oath, 60–61; medications, 68; Pedanius Dioscorides, 68; psychiatry, 63–64; surgery, 60–61; symptoms, basing treatment on, 58; syringe, hypodermic, 64; writings, medical, 65, 68

Herophilus of Chaludon, 62, 63
Hesy Re, 25–26
Hippocrates, 58–61;
Hippocratic Oath, 60–61
hospitals, 43–44, 82–83

Imhotep, 24–25, 57
India: ants used as sutures, 38–40; hospitals, 43–44; smallpox, 42–43; surgery, 36–41; Sushruta, 35, 36,

37, 39, 40; teaching aids, medical, 40–41; writings, medical, 34–36

medications, 19, 27–28, 31–32, 68, 73, 76, 83

Pedanius Dioscorides, 68
Peseshet, 27
physicians and surgeons: Alcmaeon of Croton, 62; Asclepiades of Bithynia, 63–64; Asclepius, 56–57; Charaka, 35; Claudius Galen, 74–76; Cornelius Celsus, 63, 73–74, 77–78; Erasistratus, 62, 63; experimentation on humans, 63; Herophilus of Chaludon, 62, 63; Hesy Re, 25–26; Hippocrates, 58–61; Imhotep, 24–25, 57; Pedanius Dioscorides, 68; Peseshet, 27; specialists, 26–27, 49, 52; Sushruta, 77; teaching aids for, 40–41; women as, 27; written examinations for, 52
psychiatry, 63–64
pulse, taking of, 48, 75–76

Rome: anatomy, study of, 74–75; borrowed technology, 72–73, 77; Claudius Galen, 74–76; Cornelius Celsus, 73–74, 77–78; health, public, 80–82; hospitals, 82–83; medications, 73, 76, 83; pulse, taking of, 75–76; surgery, 76–80, 82; writings, medical, 73, 75

smallpox, 42–43
Stone Age: brain surgery, 13–16, 18; medications, 19; splinting bone fractures, 18–19; superstitions, 17–18; tools, 17, 18
surgeons. *See* physicians and surgeons
surgery: abdominal, 38–40; ants used as sutures, 38–40; brain, 13–16, 18; cataract, 77–78; cesarean section, 76–77; circumcision, 28; instruments, 28, 78–80; plastic, 36–38, 82
Sushruta, 35, 77
symptoms, basing treatment on, 58
syringe, hypodermic, 64

writings, medical: *Charaka Samhita*, 35; *Chou Li*, 48, 49, 52; *De Materia Medica*, 65, 68; *De Medicina*, 73; Ebers Papyrus, 23, 24, 32; Edwin H. Smith Papyrus, 23, 24; Hippocratic Oath, 60–61; *Huang Ti Nei Ching*, 48–49, 51; Kahun Papyrus, 23–24, 31; *On Anatomical Procedure*, 75; *Sushruta Samhita*, 34–35, 36, 37, 39, 40, 77

Note: There are alternate spellings for some of the names mentioned in this book. Here are three examples:
Sushruta or Susrata or Susruta (India)
Chou or Zhou (China)
Asclepius or Asklepios (Greece)

ABOUT THE AUTHORS

Michael Woods is an award-winning science and medical writer with the Washington bureau of the *Toledo Blade* and the *Pittsburgh Post Gazette*. His articles and weekly health column, "The Medical Journal," appear in newspapers around the United States. Born in Dunkirk, New York, Mr. Woods developed a love for science and writing in childhood and studied both topics in school. His many awards include an honorary doctorate degree for helping to develop the profession of science writing. His previous work includes a children's book on Antarctica, where he has traveled on three expeditions.

Mary B. Woods is an elementary school librarian in the Fairfax County, Virginia, public school system. Born in New Rochelle, New York, Mrs. Woods studied history in college and later received a master's degree in library science. She is coauthor of a children's book on new discoveries about the ancient Maya civilization.

Photo Acknowledgments: The photographs in this book are reproduced courtesy of International Museum of Surgical Science, pp. 1, 14-15; Art Resource, NY: (Erich Lessing) pp. 2-3, 29, 59, 72, (Werner Forman Archive) pp. 21, 22-23, (Scala) pp. 70-71, 79; Corbis-Bettmann: pp. 11, 69, (Lefterhoff, Venet C. Sr.) pp. 12-13; Ancient Art & Architecture Collection, Ltd.: (Brian Wilson) p. 17, (Ronald Sheridan) pp. 25, 45, 54-55, 57, (G. Garvey) p. 80; Dinodia Picture Agency: p. 42, (D. A. Chawda) p. 33, (Milind A. Ketkar) pp. 34-35, (Isaac Kehimkar) p. 39; Christopher Liu/China Stock, pp. 46-47; Wellcome Institute Library, London, p. 48; Stock Montage, p. 50; Mary Evans Picture Library, p. 53; Science Museum/Science & Society Picture Library, p. 65; Joe McDonald/Visuals Unlimited, p. 67.

Front cover: Lori Jahnke/Hamline University Anthropology Department, left; Ancient Art & Architecture Collection, Ltd., right
Cover background: Mary Evans Picture Library